NATURAL HEALING
THROUGH
MACROBIOTICS

Natural Healing through Macrobiotics

by Michio Kushi

Foreword by Robert S. Mendelsohn, M.D.
Edited by Edward Esko *with* Marc van Cauwenberghe, M.D.

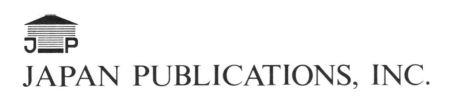

JAPAN PUBLICATIONS, INC.

Japan Publications Edition

This book was originally published under the title of *The Macrobiotic Way
of Natural Healing* by East West Foundation, 240 Washington Street,
Brookline, Massachusetts 02146.

This Japan Publications Edition is published by arrangement with East
West Foundation.

Published by
JAPAN PUBLICATIONS, INC., Tokyo and New York

Distributors:
UNITED STATES: *Kodansha America, Inc., through Farrar, Straus & Giroux, 19 Union
Square West, New York, 10003.* CANADA: *Fitzhenry & Whiteside Ltd., 195 Allstate
Parkway, Markham, Ontario, L3R 4T8.* BRITISH ISLES AND EUROPEAN CONTINENT:
Premier Book Marketing Ltd., 1 Gower Street, London WC1E 6HA. AUSTRALIA AND
NEW ZEALAND: *Bookwise International, 54 Crittenden Road, Findon, South Australia
5023.* THE FAR EAST AND JAPAN: *Japan Publications Trading Co., Ltd., 1-2-1, Sarugaku-
cho, Chiyoda-ku, Tokyo 101.*

First edition: September 1979
Twelfth printing: July 1991

LCCC No. 79-1959
ISBN 0-87040-457-1
Printed in U.S.A.

Foreword

Michio Kushi has done it again!

Following closely upon his landmark publication, *The Book of Macrobiotics*, he has now issued a powerful challenge to conventional American medicine in this new book, *Natural Healing through Macrobiotics*.

This volume appears just in time!

The past few decades have witnessed a widespread and justifiable decline of public confidence in conventional American medicine. Indeed, much of what is called "modern medicine" is now suspect of not existing at all. If one scrutinizes the six major specialties, it becomes difficult to identify, once the camouflage is removed, how much residual reality is left.

Pediatrics, my own specialty, had no more than a few thousand practitioners in the first four decades of this century, and grew hardly at all until the "Rosie the Riverters" went to work in the armament factories in World War II, providing a shot-in-the-arm to the infant formula industry. Since then, pediatricians have increased at least tenfold and infant formula sales many times that number. Without pediatric sanction, there is no way that the milk of cows and the juice of soybeans could have replaced the milk of human mothers so quickly and completely. In a major midwestern state university serving mostly the poor, the incidence of breast feeding mothers dropped from 99 % to 1 % in a ten year period. And why not, when pediatricians and their fellow travelers, nurses and social workers, handed out free commercial formula to every mother who delivered a baby. This "gift" was accompanied by the sweet lies of the physician, seducing women already pushed to work either through economic necessity or the propaganda of "fulfillment." The false assurances of these specialties lulled at least two generations of mothers into a dream world of security, enabling them to unthinkingly, but ever so trustingly expose their tender infants to the nightmare of diseases practically never found in breast fed babies (acrodermatitis enteropathica, hypocalcemic tetany, neonatal hypothyroidism, E. coli meningitis, necrotizing enterocolitis, and sudden infant death), and to insure that these infants would in later years manifest a high incidence of gastroenteritis, pneumonia, eczema, hayfever, asthma, obesity, hypertension and arteriosclerosis.

Of course, pediatricians operated with the purest of motives, but they cannot claim ignorance as an excuse. They knew the truth, since scientific studies, almost without exception, repeatedly showed the higher rates of death and illness associated with formula feedings. Then, why did they do it? Why did they tell mothers—and fathers—in honeyed words that formulas were an acceptable substitute for human milk? Why did they lead mothers and babies down the primrose path leading to such a macabre end?

The reasons are probably multiple, including greed (pediatricians and pediatrics probably could not exist without the formula manufacturers), stupidity (physicians as a group throughout history have not been noted for independence of intellect), ignorance (the multiplicity of medical journals is guaranteed to destroy communication and physicians don't stoop to reading newspapers and magazines), and misguided behavior (physicians always claim the best of intentions, while everyone knows what the road to hell is paved with).

But the reasons become relatively unimportant to those who are damaged.

The recipe for losing a pediatric practice is simple. Tell mothers the truth! Tell them bottle feeding threatens their baby's life and health. This will make the bottle-feeding mothers feel guilty (a cardinal sin in pediatrics) and they will accordingly switch doctors, leaving the truthful pediatrician with only breast-fed babies who hardly ever become ill. End of practice!

I have solved this dilemma by simply (my critics use the word "simplistically") rejecting as a patient any mother who elects not to breast feed. Other than bilateral mastectomy, there are no contraindications to breast feeding; and, given proper support, no mother is unable to breast feed. Mothers-to-be who prefer bottles are free of course to use any physician who believes formula feeding is completely compatible with good mothering. I continue to select an elite group of patients who share my own ethics and philosophy on birth, breast feeding, mothering, and large families, and whose views on other critical issues are, therefore, predictably congruent with mine. Besides, members of this "subculture" (or if you prefer, "super-culture") hardly ever get sick, thus making my own life vastly easier.

So, if pediatrics loses bottle feeding—and all the infections, allergies, illnesses and mortality associated with it—the specialty largely disappears.

The same holds for obstetrics, another specialty now in its declining years. Threatened with extinction by the falling birth rate paradoxically promoted by the "planned parenthood" activities of the OB-GYN profession itself, it survives today through abortions instead of births and through lucrative Caesarian sections instead of vaginal deliveries. Yet, the threat of rising numbers of home births and the increasing rejection of radical attitudes toward abortion forecast the disappearance of the overwhelming number of OB-GYN specialists. As healthy mothers reject stirrups, shaving, episiotomies, analgesics, routine IV fluids, monitoring, elective inductions, senseless sections, and the rest of OB technology, the result will be a diminution in the now increasing numbers of damaged and deformed infants.

Furthermore, without the irrational techniques of modern obstetrics, young obstetricians will not be able to create the clientele whose pathology enables these specialists to later emerge as mature gynecologists. Thus, Obstetrics and Gynecology joins Pediatrics as specialties that largely do not exist.

Internists would have problems even now paying the office rent without pushing "checkups," annually or more often, routinely, unthinkingly, and automatically. But the people are rapidly wising up and, as the uselessness and dangers of what has been aptly termed "the annual American fiasco" become known, Internal Medicine faces the loss of its chief source of revenue. Furthermore, increasing public skepticism of conventional medical approaches to cancer and cardiovascular disease make the status of the internist even more precarious. Having already abandoned surgery and obstetrics, the Internist joins the Pediatrician and Obstetrician-Gynecologist as another member in the category of vanishing breeds.

The surgeon may be last to go because of popular fascination, historically and now, with the drama of "going under the knife." But the four most common operations—circumcision, vasectomy, hysterectomy and tonsillectomy—seldom have scientific justification. These and other major surgical breadwinners are exposed in practically each new issue of every medical journal as not merely useless, but downright dangerous. A skeptical public now has a "show me" attitude towards cancer surgery, and the coronary bypass will soon join previous heart operations in the surgical historical museums. Surgeons are the fourth group of specialists which, like the others, soon will have to find honest work.

Psychiatry is perhaps the easiest specialty to fold its tent, because there is great doubt whether it ever in fact did exist. But regardless of its questionable origins, Thomas Szasz, Jay Ziskind, Martin Gross and a variety of others have provided the documentation that some (usually those who have been disabled by so-called "higher education," in reality merely "longer education") require to expose its non-existence, a conclusion that the less-educated citizens reached long ago by use of common sense. There are four unproven areas in psychiatry: psycho-surgery, electroshock, tranquilizers and counselling. Otherwise, it's a great specialty.

The sixth, and final, major specialty that does not exist is that of preventive medicine. This once noble endeavor, dedicated to prevent people from ever becoming patients by promotion of pure water and food supplies and adequate sewage disposal has undergone a strange transformation. A reversal has taken place. The beautiful butterfly has metamorphosed into a caterpillar. The public health officer of decades ago would not recognize his modern counterpart, hawking his wares, including risky immunizations for the prevention of mild diseases (sometimes, as in the case of the swine flu vaccine, preventing no disease at all, but causing hundreds of cases of paralysis and death) and unproven screening technology that recruits armies of new patients for doctors' offices.

Yet, the emphasis on prevention has yielded precious little in the way of results. Self examination of the breast was shown to be inadequate when thermography appeared; thermography was shown to be inadequate by X-ray mammography, which, unfortunately but predictably, caused cancers of its own. The Pap smear, with its expected incidence of false positives and false negatives, has not led to a decrease in either the incidence of cervical cancer or its death rate. But these medical toys have had one major effect, i.e., they have almost totally obscured concern with the real preventable causes of these female cancers (few pregnancies, failure to breast feed, The Pill, postmenopausal hormones).

Routine chest X-rays have lulled the public into the delusion that radiation can be trusted, thus leading to new epidemics of leukemia, thyroid cancer, and mongolism (attributed falsely to "tired eggs' of older women); while routine amniocentesis, PKU testing, blood pressure measurements, phonocardiography, and other procedures with shorter or longer names are now all suspected of resulting in a negative benefit/risk ratio.

Thus, Preventive Medicine joins Pediatrics, OB-GYN, Internal Medicine, Surgery and Psychiatry in the list of non-existent specialties.

Now, some may object, pointing out that a small minority of medical procedures are necessary and valuable. And I will quickly concede that perhaps 5% of the procedures of the Big Six Specialties has value, and therefore 5% of the specialists in these areas should be retained. After all, the problem with American medicine is that the extreme always becomes the mean. Penicillin, originally used for meningitis and severe pneumonia, becomes counter-productive when prescribed for the common cold. Cortisone, originally used for Addison's disease, becomes nightmarish when prescribed for sunburn, and I see as much hope of reversing this trend as of any other historical efforts to put the genii back in the bottle.

While the 5% *exceptions* must be noted, it remains crucial to *generalize* (although doctors are taught, with good reason for their own protection, not to make generalizations) since only by generalizing can learning and wisdom be attained.

And the generalization is that the golden age of American medicine is over. Indeed, the only way in which modern medicine can be understood is by regarding it as a religion—the religion of a secular society that has rejected its traditional value systems.

Modern medicine has at least ten of the essential components of a religion:

1. A belief system, modern medical science, which can no more be validated than the proofs of other churches of the existence of God.
2. A priestly class—the M.D.'s.
3. Temples—the hospitals
4. Acolytes and vestal maidens—nurses, social workers and para-professionals.
5. Vestments reflecting hierarchical status—the color and length of M.D.'s gowns signify their rank.
6. A rich princely class supporting the church—drug companies, insurance companies and formula houses.
7. A confessional—the history must be given truthfully to the physician.
8. An absolution—the reassuring pat on the back—"you're fine, come back next year."
9. Selling of indulgences—the outrageous fees, likely to bring down this modern church just as it did the medieval church.
10. Similarity of language—I have confidence in my plumber, but "I have *faith* in my doctor; the doctor-patient relationship is "sacred."

Once medicine is regarded as no more than—and no less than—a religious system, it can then be treated as such, and compared with other religious healing systems. Unfortunately, the religion of modern medicine proves to be worship of a god who fails to answer, who is powerless and who, in fact, deceives. This, of course, is the definition of idolatry, and in this context all of modern medicine becomes understandable.

The false god of modern medicine even goes so far as to require, like his predecessor gods of heathen religions thousands of years ago, child sacrifices. The ancient Moloch of those idolatries demanded that parents, in order to insure successful crops, pass their children through physical fire. The modern Moloch similarly demands that parents pass chemical fire (heat-sterilized formula) through their children. The purpose is similar—infant formula insures that mothers and fathers can both go to work to achieve sustenance and success. Scientific studies as well as historical evidence clearly prove the sacrifice of life and health resulting from infant formula compared to breast milk, and only the approval of the physician-priest enables mothers and fathers to equate cows' milk to human milk. Indeed, were physicians to behave according to the standards of science and honesty, formula feeding a baby would doubtless be considered child abuse.

A large part of the reason for the failure of the religion of modern medicine lies in the unwillingness to seriously address itself to nutritional concerns. (Perhaps this is due in part to the Christian tradition, stated by Matthew and others, that what comes out of the mouth is more important than what goes in.) In any case, as the religion of modern medicine loses its power and influence, its former adherents must seek other, more valid, religious systems. Some will turn to the medical teachings of Christian Science and Jehovah's Witnesses. Jews will rediscover their traditional medical teachings emphasizing nutrition, from the Old Testament through Talmudic and Maimonidean medicine, and culminating in the contemporary medical ethical teachings of Jakobovits, Rosner, Feldman, Bleich, Soloveichik and others.

In this context, the universalist Macrobiotic approach to life demands close examination, particularly by Western physicians and patients who are almost totally ignorant not only of its content, but even of its very existence. Kushi's present volume provides and unparalleled opportunity for Western-trained physicians to discover the time-tested diagnostic and therapeutic approaches of a rich culture thus far closed to them.

Kushi gives detailed descriptions of diseases of various organ-systems (digestive, respiratory, circulatory, lymphatic, nervous, reproductive), with particular emphasis on natural pregnancy and childbirth at the one end of life and cancer nearer the other,.

As might be expected, much of his teaching is at sharp variance with American medicine:

1. Rather than depending on "scientific nutrition," he teaches "study the traditional dietary customs of the people who have been living there for thousands of years." Sensible, isn't it?
2. Rather than depend on deodorants, he teaches "unpleasant body odor is nothing but the result of a diet high in meat and other animal products, as well as in various types of dairy products."
3. On the etiology of cancer, "since the more yin foods . . . are consumed widely in Japan, the people in that nation suffer from stomach cancer to a much greater degree than in America . . ."
4. The sections of hematology—including the origin of blood, and the treatments of leukemia and pernicious anemia—cry out for the attention of modern hematologists.
5. "Hemophilia can be relieved through macrobiotics, but it may take several years."
6. "It is possible to change your blood type" is a statement likely to chill the blood of western-trained physicians.
7. "If you are a vegetarian, you should not develop appendicitis." The macrobiotic approach to acute appendicitis begins, not with surgery, but with a 2 or 3 day fast and cold applications.
8. As far as hernia is concerned, "the only way to relieve this condition is to cause the organs to contract through eating. By eating the standard macrobiotic way, a hernia can be relieved in four to six months." The same genre of prescription applies to hay fever, stuttering, snoring and bad breath.
9. For pneumonia, "if you can obtain a live carp, first offer your thanks and appreciation to it, and after killing it, extract a small quantity of its blood . . ." and the detailed treatment continues.
10. On length of labor,"Among macrobiotic women . . . the average is between

      8 and 10 hours for the first child and 4 and 8 hours for the following children," about half as long as in others.

11. I am happy to read Kushi's opposition to silver nitrate in newborns' eyes, which causes a chemical inflammation possibly responsible for myopia, astigmatism and other refraction problems later.

12. He is also opposed to artificial formula and glucose solutions given to newborns.

13. "Among cancers, breast cancer is one of the easiest to relieve through macrobiotics as are uterine and skin cancer . . . . Operations or radiation treatments are unnecessary for these conditions and should be avoided."

14. If a mother develops a breast cyst or tumor, "she should continue nursing with the affected breast. This will further speed the relief of her condition."

15. Regarding appendectomies, "it is also a contributing factor in the development of multiple sclerosis," The same is true of hysterectomy.

16. "Parkinson's disease can be relieved in anywhere from one to six months."

Western physicians can be expected to react to macrobiotic medicine with the usual name-calling, and Kushi advocates by now are used to epithets such as "quacks, nuts, extremists, faddists, fakes and enthusiasts." But this automatic response doesn't work any more, since the medical advocates of "better living through chemistry" have lost their magical power over the people.

In these twilight years of death-oriented, run-away medical technology, the macrobiotic approach to disease and healing comes like a breath of fresh air. Of the hundreds of publications on health and disease that have passed over my desk for review in the past few decades, this book provides the most important alternative to our rapidly failing system of western medicine.

Kushi's latest volume is must reading for every physician, and I will know that America's medical schools have reached maturity when *Natural Healing Through Macrobiotics* becomes part of the standard curriculum.

Meanwhile, patients can't afford to wait for their busy doctors to learn about this apparently new, but in reality centuries-old system. People need practical and realistic help now and this highly readable volume, filled with fascinating hypotheses, good knowledge of modern medicine, profound wisdom, enjoyable humor and a large dose of justifiable optimism is, in my judgment, a vital key to good health and life.

This book on Macrobiotic Medicine, destined to have a profound effect on our nation's future, merits top priority by every citizen.

ROBERT S. MENDELSOHN, M.D.

Associate Professor, Department of Preventive Medicine and Community Health, Abraham Lincoln School of Medicine, University of Illinois; *Nationally syndicated columnist*, "The People's Doctor"; *Medical Director*, American International Hospital, Zion, Illinois; *Formerly, National Director*, Medical Consultation Service, Project Head Start; *Formerly, Chairman*, Medical Licensure Committee, State of Illinois

Preface

Every spring the young shoots of green leaves give me great joy and surprise. This spring my husband's book, *Natural Healing through Macrobiotics*, blossomed out, and I am very grateful for the efforts of our many friends who worked together to complete this book. There was much work behind the scenes—making tapes, transcribing them, and editing them to produce the study reports and the *Order of the Universe* magazine. Then, the students compiled all that material, edited it again, and put it into finished form as a book. I can't count the number of friends whose activities and warm, sincere energies went into this one book on macrobiotic healing.

George Ohsawa first introduced to the modern world the traditional, natural ways of macrobiotic healing and oriental medicine, beginning in Japan almost 40 years ago and also teaching in Western countries, especially in France. He was our teacher, and because of him we have a happy life. When I was staying at George Ohsawa's World Government Study House in 1950, one of his strongest wishes was to send a number of his students, at least 12, from Japan to foreign countries. This was right after World War II, and Japan was in great confusion. The Japanese currency was practically worthless abroad. It was almost impossible for ordinary people to go out from Japan; only a few governmental people could travel. Nevertheless Mr. Ohsawa encouraged his students to this adventure. He called it the "Great Escape"—literally, from Japan—but the real meaning was an escape to freedomland for the real life of challenging adventures.

On February 3, 1950, when I first came to George Ohsawa's study house, my future husband was already in the United States. He was the first "escapee" among the students. Mr. Ohsawa called him the "number one young ambassador of world government." Mr. Ohsawa spoke of Michio many times in his lectures, almost every day. He told us Michio had graduated from his school, Maison Ignoramus, after a total of only 48 hours' study; how smart he was, how Michio's mother was different from ordinary mothers, and so on. He always advised everyone to follow Michio's example and escape like him as soon as possible—better yet, at once. That was the way he finished most of his lectures.

But Mr. Ohsawa was also worried about Michio because he didn't have much experience in macrobiotic practice yet, and also he had a tendency toward a weak heart and lungs. After a 13-day trip crossing the Pacific Ocean by boat, Michio had reached San Francisco on Thanksgiving Day 1949; but he did not send any letters for almost four months after he left Japan. Then one day in April of 1950, when the cherry blossoms were almost gone, George Ohsawa brought Michio's letter to his morning lecture. Mr. Ohsawa was almost jumping and dancing. He told us that Michio had finally reached New York. Michio's letter was very beautiful, and Mr. Ohsawa read it at the lecture like a reading of poetry. That letter captured me for the rest of my life!

The study house was located in Hiyoshi, outside Tokyo. From there, many students went out to foreign countries to begin spreading macrobiotics, when George Ohsawa was still in his early 50's: Mr. Tomio Kikuchi, to Brazil; Mr. and Mrs. Herman Aihara, to the West Coast of the United States; Mr. Clim Yoshimi, to France; Mr. Roland Yasuhara, to Spain; Mr. Ave Nakamura, to Germany; Shizuko Yamamoto, to New York; Mr. Junsei Yamazaki, to California to help in the establishment of Chico San; and several others.

My husband was lecturing here and there throughout America from the beginning, but the first time we organized a summer camp ourselves was in 1965 on Martha's Vineyard. At that time, many other students of George Ohsawa were beginning their teaching activities in other countries. George Ohsawa came from Europe to teach at our summer camp. He was so happy to see us; we sat with him on the sands of beautiful Martha's Vineyard Island, and dreamed together of the future peaceful world for which we were all working.

When Mr. Ohsawa died suddenly on April 24, 1966, his passing made a dramatic turning point in our lives. From that time on my husband put all his effort and energy into giving lectures. He didn't mind if it was a rainy day or a snowy day; he lectured usually two times a week, and sometimes several times a week. It almost seemed as if he gave the lectures for himself. He did not mind how many people attended; in the beginning, sometimes only a handful of people came. He went on in the selfless spirit of a samurai practicing to perfect his swordmanship.

In the beginning, we never advertised or made any effort to attract students. We don't know how they knew, but more and more people were knocking on our door. Most of them were young; this was toward the beginning of the so-called "hippy" era. So, paradoxically enough, just as LSD and marijuana were beginning to become popular in this country, we were beginning our educational efforts. All of the students were fairly eager to seek a new way of life, but they were rather like drifting leaves, floating about on the winds or the waves. The purpose of my husband's lectures was to change their total way of life; so the contents of each lecture depended on the student's conditions or their wishes. His teaching method was not like the systematized curriculum of a school course, but covered a whole range of academic and also practical subjects: oriental philosophy, oriental medicine, oriental culture, Bible study, history, diet, women and children's studies, natural birth and education in general, household organization and care, ancient and modern science, chemistry, shiatsu massage, palm healing, dō-in, acupuncture, astrology and astronomy, meditation and exercise, new political and economic systems as well as the new vision of the future world—he introduced everything. Starting at that time he has put his whole effort into lecturing; helping young people launch businesses in the natural foods area; and establishing the movement in this country towards natural organic food and natural way of life.

The present book is based on many of these lectures that covered the basic principles of medicine and health. To transcribe and organize the seminar material into book form has involved the efforts of many people. We very much appreciate the work of Edward Esko, Marc Van Cauwenberghe, and all of the others who have contributed to its completion. Edward Esko is one of our most steady friends, who has been continuously devoting himself to the ongoing activities of the East West Foundation; Marc Van Cauwenberghe is a medical doctor and one of the most promising contributors to the future of medicine, curing many serious illnesses through the application of the macrobiotic way.

We should be aware that there are no fixed medicinal regimens on which we can always depend—certainly not the "medicine" promoted by television advertising: aspirin, bufferin, nose drops, and so on! Medicine cannot be standardized; it must be tailor-made to fit everyone's personal differences. Only you are able to do this for yourself and your family. To cure sickness requires tremendous patience, but if you take full responsibility to do that yourself, you will be surprised at the simple ways you can discover to solve your problems.

I think the most important thing is to realize deeply that we cannot depend upon anyone else for our well-being; we must take full responsibility for our own health and for that of our families. Several times when our children have become sick, because of that feeling of responsibility, fortunately, we have been able to discover the proper course of healing and to pass through those times successfully.

We also need to be very careful to take care of ourselves *before* any symptoms arise. It is very difficult to restore health *after* someone's physical condition has become so unbalanced that symptoms of sickness appear; then, we are forced to look around for special treatments. Day-to-day observation of our condition and our family's condition is essential to maintain health and prevent sickness from developing. Of course, we should not have an anxious attitude, but we should be carefully observant.

Simply reading this book will not tell you everything you need to know in order to take care of sickness, but I can say with assurance that it contains more information about the ways of healing than I have had to deal with in over 25 years of macrobiotic living. It can serve as a basis for your study and practice of healing; however, without our own observations and careful judgment of our varying conditions, this general knowledge cannot be effective. We must fully participate with real understanding of a person's individual condition and habits. Therefore, you should not depend upon this information alone: the most important thing is, how you use it.

In my opinion this book is a stepping-stone that can help you develop a deeper understanding for your life. It is my hope that you will use this knowledge to create health and happiness in your own life, and to help many other people to do the same.

AVELINE TOMOKO KUSHI
Brookline, Massachusetts
May 1978

Acknowledgments

I would like to extend my deep appreciation to all of those who assisted in the creation of this book, which is based on the seminars and lectures presented by Michio Kushi at the East West Foundation in Boston. The task of recording, transcribing, and editing the spoken material presented by Mr. Kushi has involved the cooperation of a number of people. Much of the material in this book was taken from a seminar on *Disease: Origin, Causes, and Cures* presented by Michio Kushi during November and December, 1972. I wish to thank Miss Joan Mansolilli for her patient work in recording and transcribing this material, as well as Mr. Dale McNutt for recording and reproducing the many accompanying diagrams and illustrations.

I would also like to thank my collaborator, Dr. Marc Van Cauwenberghe, of Ghent, Belgium, for his invaluable assistance in recording and transcribing Mr. Kushi's seminar on *The Natural Macrobiotic Approach to Major Modern Illnesses* presented in May, 1977, and also for his patience in reviewing the text from a medical point of view.

This book would not have been possible without the assistance of Miss Olivia Oredson, who, from the very beginning of the project in May 1977, contributed her time and energy. She has helped in the typing and coordination of every phase of the manuscript, from her initial suggestion that the Foundation publish a book on Natural Healing to the composing of the final text.

I would also like to thank Mr. Sherman Goldman, editor of the *East West Journal*, and Mr. Phillip Jannetta, editor of the *Order of the Universe*, for reviewing the text and for suggesting additional modifications and improvements.

I would also like to thank Mr. Tim Goodwin, Peter and Bonnie Harris, Mr. Stephen Uprichard, Miss Teresa Turner, and other members of the Foundation staff for their guidance and assistance, as well as Mrs. Aveline Kushi and Dr. Robert Mendelsohn for their introductory comments and continuing support and guidance. I would also like to thank my wife, Wendy, for her patience and support during the long months that this book was written, and extend my heartfelt appreciation on behalf of the staff and many friends of the East West Foundation to Mr. David Hinckle of Earthbeam Natural Foods in Burlingame, California, for his encouragement and support.

Finally, I would like to express my sincere gratitude and appreciation to Michio Kushi, George Ohsawa, and all others who have pursued the dream of a healthy and happy world.

EDWARD ESKO

Introduction

Not long ago, I was visited by a young woman who I will call "Beth." Beth had been experiencing irregularities with her menstruation, along with a persistent, growing pain in her lower back, and facial blemishes. A medical examination revealed that she had developed a cyst, about the size of an orange, in one of her ovaries. Her doctor had advised exploratory surgery, with the likelihood that the tumor and perhaps the ovary itself would be removed.

I felt that the problem was caused by an improper balance in her daily diet, particularly the overconsumption of dairy products. During her visit, I recommended that she begin the macrobiotic way of eating, along with the application of several simple external treatments that could be easily prepared at home. To the surprise of both Beth and her doctor, the cyst was no longer detectable after six weeks of practicing this regime. Her physician, a well-known gynecologist, remarked that in all her years of practice, she had never seen a case such as this.

During more than seven years of study and practice of the macrobiotic way of natural healing, I have had the opportunity to witness hundreds of cases, involving a variety of illnesses, which have had a similar outcome to the case of Beth. Although less dramatic than Beth's, my own experience with macrobiotic healing began in the late 1960's when I was student at Temple University in Philadelphia. It was during this time that I started to seek a more comprehensive understanding of life and the universe through the study of the traditional wisdom of the Orient.

My search began with the wisdom of Vedanta, proceeded through Taoism and Chinese thought, and then led on to Zen and Shintoism. I discovered the macrobiotic teachings of George Ohsawa at this time, and soon realized that macrobiotics offered the means of actually transforming this timeless wisdom of the Orient into a living reality. Through macrobiotics, I came to understand that the enlightenment that I had been searching for had been directly in front of me all along, literally as close as my next meal. As I adopted the macrobiotic lifestyle based on natural law, the allergies I had suffered from since childhood began to disappear, my eyes became bright and clear, I lost excessive weight, and my outlook grew more positive and happy.

In 1972, I moved to Boston from Philadelphia in order to deepen my understanding of macrobiotic healing through study and association with Michio Kushi and others. Since 1973, I have been closely associated with the East West Foundation, an experience which has afforded many opportunities for further study and practical application, including the chance to have taught and lectured throughout the United States, as well as in England and Belgium, and to have edited the *Order of the Universe*, the *Case History Report*, and other publications dealing with macrobiotics and natural healing. During this period I have advised several hundred people about the way of health and happiness through macrobiotics.

Through these and other experiences, I have come to realize that health, happiness, and freedom are actually the natural human condition, and are far easier to achieve and maintain than their opposite states. If we live in harmony with our natural environment, health and happiness will follow automatically. My observations and direct experiences with the effects of food on our physical condition and mental outlook have convinced me that the most basic and fundamental way of achieving health and happiness is to begin selecting, preparing, and eating our daily meals in accordance with the order of nature. This universal, common sense method is freely available to everyone, regardless of age, sex, race, occupation, religion, or nationality. All that is required is a desire to enjoy a life free from sickness, disease, and unhappiness, along with the wish to claim the human birthright of a free, happy, and healthy life.

The age of "dietary anarchy" now prevails throughout modern society. Traditional patterns of eating—based around whole cereal grains and cooked vegetables as the staple foods—which were followed for thousands of years throughout the world have been abandoned in favor of the modern diet consisting of large quantities of animal food; heavily refined and processed flour and grain; refined sugar; dairy products; fruits and spices imported from great distances; chemicalized, industrialized and artificial foods; and powerful drugs and medications. Not only is this modern way of eating widespread in the industrial nations in both East and West, but it is being exported at an increasingly rapid rate throughout the world. As a result, in spite of the great prosperity brought on by technological advances, we are in the midst of a biological Noah's Flood which is reflected in the increasing worldwide incidence of degenerative diseases such as cancer, heart disease, mental illness, etc., along with an epidemic of social ailments such as divorce, drug abuse, juvenile delinquency, crime, and the ever-present possibility of nuclear war.

More than forty years ago, Dr. Alexis Carrel, a Nobel Prize winning physiologist at the Rockefeller Institute, foresaw our present situation and, in his book *Man the Unknown*, proposed a complete re-evaluation of our approach to life, the universe, and ourselves. In the preface to his comprehensive volume we read:

> Before beginning this work the author realized its difficulty, its almost impossibility. He undertook it merely because somebody had to undertake it, because men cannot follow modern civilization along its present course, because they are degenerating. They have been fascinated by the beauty of the science of inert matter. They have not understood that their body and consciousness are subjected to natural laws, more obscure than, but as inexorable as, the laws of the sidereal world. Neither have they understood that they cannot transgress these laws without being punished. They must, therefore, learn the necessary relations of the cosmic universe, of their fellow men, and of their inner selves, and also those of their tissues and their mind. Indeed, man stands above all things. Should he degenerate, the beauty of civilization, and even the grandeur of the physical universe, would vanish. For these reasons this book was written.

The natural laws of which Dr. Carrel wrote are expressed in macrobiotics as the principle of dualistic monism: yin changes into yang, and yang changes into yin, everywhere and forever. The greatest and most grandiose civilizations have all experienced eventual decline and decay. Nothing is exempt from this most fundamental law. At the same time, however, within the potential Armageddon of modern civilization, the seeds of the biological, psychological and spiritual restoration of humanity are beginning to grow, just as the depth of winter produces spring, and the peak of night leads to dawn.

Over the past fifty years, the most fundamental way to achieve this restoration has been taught throughout the world as the understanding and practice of macrobiotics. When Michio Kushi graduated from Tokyo University more than twenty-seven years ago, prior to coming to the United States for graduate study at Columbia, his interest in world peace through world federal government led him to investigate the work of George Ohsawa. Mr. Ohsawa proposed that only with the biological reconstruction of humanity on an individual basis through the basic means of daily life and diet, could world peace be established. Observation of the human condition for close to twenty-five years had led Mr. Ohsawa to this insight. His conclusions are contained in three basic works available in English: *Zen Macrobiotics*, *The Book of Judgement*, and *The Macrobiotic Guidebook to Living*. Inspired by this view of life, Mr. Kushi has been teaching, writing, and lecturing throughout the United States, Canada, Western Europe, and the Far East, in order to further the understanding and practical application of this traditional way of life based on harmony with the order of the universe for the goal of world peace. Many of his conclusions are contained in *The Book of Macrobiotics—The Universal Way of Health and Happiness* published by Japan Publications, Inc. in 1977.

Since 1965, Mr. Kushi has centered his educational activities in the Boston area, where thousands of students from throughout the United States and the world have come to study. Many of these students have subsequently begun enterprises making the macrobiotic way of life easily available for all. As a result, numerous outlets for the distribution of high quality natural and organic foods have been established in America. These include Erewhon, which, in addition to having several retail outlets in New England, with an affiliate in Southern California, also provides natural and organic products to several hundreds of retail stores in North America. Among the many macrobiotic restaurants established by these students, the Seventh Inn and Sanae restaurants in Boston are perhaps the leading examples.

In 1971, a 12-page newsletter was started by several of Mr. Kushi's students. Since then, the *East West Journal* has grown to become a 96-page monthly news magazine with an international readership of 120,000. The *East West Journal* regularly publishes articles by, and interviews with, leading contemporary philosophical, social and scientific thinkers working in their respective fields to express the unifying principle in Western terms.

In 1972, Mr. and Mrs. Kushi established the East West Foundation for One Peaceful World. It is a federally approved, nonprofit educational and cultural institution, created for the purpose of implementing a sound and human technology for the biological, social and spiritual development of all people. The activities of the Foundation now include education, publication, cultural and student exchange, the development of agricultural and educational centers, and research.

In 1977, the Michio Kushi Institute was established in London to provide systematic programs in macrobiotics and natural healing. In the following year, the Kushi Institute was established in the Boston area as well. Mr. Kushi's activities for the benefit of society at large also include plans for the presentation of regional Congresses of macrobiotics in Europe, North and South America and the Far East, to be followed by the *World Congress of Macrobiotics* during the coming decade.

The overall aim of macrobiotic healing extends beyond the relief of individual sickness to the eventual realization of a peaceful and harmonious world society. This goal, toward which so many of history's greatest philosophers, thinkers, and teachers have dedicated their lives, will be realized at last as an increasing number of people begin to apply the order of nature to their daily lives. A healthy nation is composed of healthy communities, which are in turn the natural outcome of strong and healthy families. The basis of family health and happiness is the understanding and ability of each member to take responsibility for and successfully manage his or her own total health. It is our hope that this book may serve as a practical guide for the achievement of that goal, the basic aim of macrobiotics.

Macrobiotic healing is based on the development and maintenance of a dynamic balance between the two primary tendencies found in the universe. Thus, with a simple scale used for measuring weight, balance is achieved by placing equal amounts of material on either side. If one side contains less weight, it will begin to rise, as the heavier side sinks. The side which falls does so as a result of the influence of downward, or centripetal force, while the other side rises because of the influence of centrifugal, or expanding force.

These two basic forces, known in the Orient as yin and yang, are universal tendencies which govern all phenomena. For example, on the earth, we are constantly receiving an incoming, downward force from the sun, stars, planets, and the constellations, which pushes everything onto the surface of the planet and causes the earth to turn and revolve around the sun. At the same time, the earth, because of its rotation, generates an opposite, expanding or outgoing force. The interplay between these two forces—centripetality, or yang, and centrifugality, or yin—creates all manifestations on our planet and throughout the universe.

In this book, the downward, centripetal force is described as heaven's force, while the opposite, expanding force is referred to as the force of earth. Each movement creates respective physical tendencies. For example, centripetal, or yang ($\triangle$) force creates contraction, density, heaviness, rapid motion and high temperature. Centrifugal, or yin ($\triangledown$) force creates expansion, diffusion, lightness, slower motion and low temperature. Also, at their extreme, each force changes into its opposite, as high temperature causes expansion and low temperature results in contraction. Yin and yang are not static conditions but rather tendencies which cycle continually or change into each other as is obvious in the sequence of day changing into night and then night giving way to the day. The progression from winter to summer and then back to winter is another example of the interplay of opposites that governs all life.

Health is the natural result of maintaining a dynamic balance of yin and yang in our daily eating and life style. An understanding of the laws that govern these two antagonistic, yet complementary tendencies can unlock the secrets of the human body and its relation to the surrounding environment. It can lead to the realization of our origin and destiny as human beings. I hope that you will explore through the chapters of this book, the wonderful order of nature and the marvelous workings of the human body, for the purpose of achieving health, happiness, and infinite freedom.

EDWARD ESKO
Brookline, Massachusetts
April 1978

Contents

Foreword *by Robert S. Mendelsohn, M.D.* 5
Preface *by Aveline Tomoko Kushi* 11
Acknowledgments 15
Introduction *by Edward Esko* 17

1. **The Way of Natural Healing** 23
   The Stages of Sickness 24
   The Seven Levels of Eating 27

2. **The Progressive Development of Sickness** 29
   The Standard Way of Macrobiotic Eating 29
   The Modern Diet 32
   A Nutritional Approach to Cancer 33

3. **The Way of Diagnosis** 49
   Appendix 80

4. **The Digestive System** 83
   The Physiology of Digestion 83
   The Macrobiotic Approach to Digestive Diseases 86
   Appendix 93

5. **The Respiratory System** 95
   The Macrobiotic Approach to Respiratory Diseases 95
   Appendix 101

6. **The Circulatory and Lymphatic Systems** 103
   The Blood 103
   The Macrobiotic Approach to Blood Diseases 104
   The Circulatory System 110
   The Macrobiotic Approach to Cardiovascular Diseases 111
   The Lymphatic System 113
   The Macrobiotic Approach to Diseases of the Lymphatic System 114
   Appendix 115

7. **The Endocrine System** 119
   The General Pattern of the Endocrine System 119
   The Physiology of the Endocrine System 121
   A Summary of the Endocrine System 124
   Diseases of the Endocrine Glands 125

The Macrobiotic Approach to Endocrine Diseases   127
Diabetes Mellitus   129
Hyperinsulinism   132

8. **The Nervous System   135**
Consciousness and Communication   138
The Macrobiotic Approach to Multiple Sclerosis and Other Diseases of the
Nervous System   142

9. **The Reproductive System   153**
The Male Reproductive System   153
Diseases of the Male Reproductive System   153
The Female Reproductive System   155
Diseases of the Female Reproductive System   158
Venereal Diseases   161

10. **The Face and Head   163**
The Macrobiotic Approach to Eye Diseases   163
The Macrobiotic Approach to Ear Diseases   167
The Teeth   168
The Hair   171

11. **Natural Pregnancy, Childbirth, and Childcare   173**
Pregancy   173
The Stages of Pregnancy   173
Embryonic Education (Tai-Kyo)   174
Disorders Which May Arise During Pregnancy   176
Childbirth   176
The Newborn Baby   179
Food and the Stages of Human Development   182
The Macrobiotic Approach to Children's Diseases   184

Appendix A: *Natural Applications   187*
Appendix B: *Arthritis   191*
Appendix C: *Principles of the Order of the Universe   193*
Bibliography *195*
Index *199*

CHAPTER ONE

The Way of Natural Healing

In this volume, we hope to illustrate how an understanding of the cause, mechanism, and relief of the major illnesses experienced by modern man can lead to an understanding of life itself. First, however, let us review the current health picture in the United States.

It is now estimated that one out of four people in America will eventually develop cancer, and this rate is increasing rapidly. Most of us have no idea of what cancer is, not to mention an understanding of what causes it or how it can be prevented or cured. Every year, ten million cases of heart disease are reported, while an additional ten million go unreported. According to recent statistics, there are about 250,000 automobile accidents in America every year, which result in about 50,000 deaths. These often occur because many people have lost their natural coordination and intuition. Ninety-seven percent of the adult population in this country will develop some form of arthritis or rheumatism, while millions more suffer from allergies, diabetes, sexual problems, and a variety of mental and emotional disorders.

Most of us in this country have at least two colds each year, meaning that there are at least 400 million colds annually in the United States alone. At present, we do not understand what a cold is or how to cure it.

Modern medicine has developed to the point where it is now able to relieve symptoms. For example, if cancer develops in the stomach, one approach is to remove part of this organ, after which the cancer is often considered to be cured. The same is true of infectious diseases, for which the practice of vaccination is recommended. Vaccination is the injection of a small quantity of bacteria, which causes a person to develop a mild case of the disease. This does not eliminate the cause of the disease, however.

We must realize that, as modern people, we are ignorant of what life and health really are. When it comes to the most fundamental questions of life, we are now in the midst of what we might call the "age of ignorance." Three to four thousand years of development have demonstrated that our present direction will not necessarily produce solutions. We must now re-evaluate our present orientation and way of thinking, including our understanding of man and the universe.

Many people are turning to macrobiotic medicine, which can be thought of as the medicine of the universe. The aim of medicine of this type is to help each individual live harmoniously with nature and the surrounding environment. In this way, each person is encouraged to achieve his or her own status as a healthy human being. Macrobiotic medicine aims at more than just the relief of individual symptoms, being equally concerned with the establishment of health, peace, and freedom on a family, community, national, and even global scale.

We can summarize the principles of macrotiotic healing as follows:

1. Understand the orderliness of nature.   We are presently witnessing the possible end of modern civilization as a result of deep-seated chronic biological degeneration. By the time the present generation of children become adult, this dramatic tragedy may very well take place. To confirm this, one need only refer to the statistics documenting the steady increase in cancer, heart disease, multiple sclerosis, deafness, and a multitude of other physical and mental disorders. However, this course is not irreversible. Once we self-reflect and decide to take positive steps to change ourselves, this tragic situation can be turned into its opposite, both for individuals, and for society as a whole. Therefore, the most primary method for avoiding this potential tragedy is not any particular technique, including dietary adjustment, but self-reflection. If we can first realize that all of our sickness and unhappiness have resulted from nothing but our own mistakes and improper judgment, and then resolve to change, we can very easily turn our direction into one of continuing health and happiness.

2. *Our view should be comprehensive.* Today, the study of the body is called physiology, whereas the study of the mind is called psychology, and both are considered as separate sciences. Further, each organ or part of the body is given separate consideration, and a whole field of specialists are created for each. For example, if a person develops ear trouble, he or she will go to an ear specialist. However, the ears are organically related to other parts of the body, and trouble with these organs means that other parts of the body are also not functioning properly. People with skin disorders are advised to see a skin specialist, but this approach often overlooks the deeper internal disorders which produce skin disease, such as malfunction of the liver, the inability of the kidneys to smoothly discharge excess, or intestinal and digestive disfunction.

At present, we are in the midst of a rapid deterioration of the biological, psychological, and spiritual quality of humanity, which is reflected in the steady increase in the incidence of degenerative disease, mental illness, and social disharmony. In order to change this course, we must now re-evaluate our present orientation. Rather than continuing to further subdivide and analyze, our approach to healing should be based on a comprehensive view of man's relationship with the universe. Naturally, the techniques which develop from this understanding should be simple, practical, and easily understood by everyone. In fact, the process of developing and maintaining health should not be separate from the normal, day-to-day process of life itself.

The Stages of Sickness

Sickness is nothing but the result of being out of balance with nature and the universe. It usually develops through the following general stages:

1. **Fatigue or Tiredness.** This includes both physical and mental fatigue. A person who frequently changes his job, place of living, or spouse, is suffering from this stage of sickness. When healthy people work very hard, they may naturally feel exhausted, but, after a good night's sleep, they will awaken the next morning feeling completely refreshed and eager for any challenge or difficulty. This is quite different from the chronic fatigue which many people presently experience.

Try gripping your shoulder tightly, and also the back of your neck. If you feel pain, then you have the tendency to suffer from chronic fatigue. The major causes of this prevalent problem in the modern world are lack of physical exercise plus over-eating and over-drinking, in particular the consumption of meat and sugar, all of which tax the muscles and circulation.

2.   Aches and Pains.   Problems such as muscle aches, occasional headaches, menstrual cramps, stomach pains, and others occur at this second stage, in which the nervous system is starting to weaken.

3.   Blood Diseases.   Sicknesses of the blood are often the result of a chronically over-acid blood condition, or of a fatty, sticky, or cholesterol-filled bloodstream. The quality of everyone's blood is different. If the condition of the blood is chronically poor, illnesses such as anemia, leukemia, asthma, hemophilia, jaundice, varicose veins, mononucleosis, skin diseases, leprosy, and others can easily occur.

   Unfortunately, many of these sicknesses as considered incurable. However, even a sickness as serious as leukemia is relatively easy to control through proper eating, even if the person has suffered from it for several years.

4.   Emotional Disorders.   This category includes problems such as irritability, impatience, upset, anger, anxiety, worry, fear, and uneasiness. A healthy person is not bothered by negative emotional states. If we become angry even once a year, we are not completely healthy. Ideally, we should not become angry even once during an entire lifetime.

5.   Organ Diseases.   Tuberculosis, heart disease, diabetes, emphysema, ulcers, cirrhosis of the liver, and gallstones are examples of organ sicknesses. At this stage, the organs are starting to degenerate.

6.   Nerve Diseases.   These include various types of mental illness, multiple sclerosis, spinal meningitis, Parkinson's disease, and different types of paralysis. Problems with the peripheral nerves are included in this category, as are disorders such as dull responses to others, forgetfulness, and social crimes.

7.   Arrogance.   This occurs when we try to separate ourselves from nature and the universe, and happens in one of two ways. The first is yang arrogance, and it appears in the form of a domineering, conquering, or self-insistent personality which tends to drive others away. The second type of arrogance is generally more yin. Persons who are exclusive or who confine themselves suffer from arrogance of this type. Often, when friends offer help or advice, a person with yin arrogance will refuse to listen and will withdraw. Many elderly people have this problem, as do many who consider themselves to be devout or religious. This type of person is usually not open to the opinions or suggestions of others.

   Arrogance is actually the underlying cause of all human sickness and unhappiness, and is at the same time the end point of the first six stages. Ultimately, all people who suffer from arrogance commit suicide by dying an unnatural death, either through sickness, war, accident, or other causes. The basic purpose of macrobiotic healing is to cure arrogance. Even though modern medicine can relieve a variety of symptoms, as can acupuncture and other forms of oriental medicine, it cannot cure this basic disease of arrogance.

Illnesses can also be classified as diseases of adjustment or degenerative sicknesses. Stages one to four of the above categories can be classified as adjustment sicknesses, while stages five through seven are degenerative.

1. Sicknesses of Adjustment. This type of sickness often occurs after someone who has been eating good food for some time suddenly eats something bad, and develops diarrhea, stomach pains, fever, or vomiting. Symptoms like these are often considered sicknesses, but in fact, are nothing but discharges of poisons or toxins. Another example is tonsilitis, which occurs when the lymphatic system tries to localize toxins which have entered the body through improper food. In this case, the accompanying fever is simply an attempt to "burn off" this excess. Through adjustments such as these, we maintain a more neutral or balanced condition.

Often, when a woman eats unbalanced food, her menstruation will become irregular. This is another example of an adjustment sickness. Also, people who eat meat and other animal foods often experience an unpleasant body odor. Again, this is nothing but a discharge of excess, as are many skin diseases, headaches, and discharges of various types. Most of the time, it is better not to interfere with a sickness of this type unless it is very acute, as in the case of a very high fever, for which special treatments are necessary. Once the excess has been discharged, the symptoms will usually disappear. If you continue to eat well during this process, your body will remain strong and your self-healing abilities will develop. Adjustments such as these should not be considered as actual sicknesses.

2. Degenerative Sicknesses. Degenerative ailments should be considered as actual sicknesses, since they result from the chronic deterioration of various bodily organs and functions. Some forms of degenerative illness arise when the body's cells begin to decompose into their primitive, pre-cellular form. Cells are originally formed by the aggregation and fusion of millions of bacteria, and when the reverse process occurs, we call this an infectious disease.

A heart murmur resulting from improper coordination of the cardiac muscle represents another type of degenerative sickness, as is kidney malfunction resulting from excessive fluid intake. Another type of degenerative condition results from the repeated intake of refined sugar, which produces a chronically over-acid bloodstream. This causes a chronic degeneration in the quality of the bones and teeth. Diseases such as epilepsy, cancer, and diabetes are also included in this category.

If a person who has been eating properly for several years eats a hamburger, he will often vomit or have diarrhea soon afterward. This arises because the hamburger is not a natural human food. As our condition improves through proper eating, we become increasingly sensitive to the effects of food. If we don't experience some type of reaction after eating bad food, we are accumulating excess and our condition is degenerating. The external symptoms of this may not appear for twenty years, but our bodily functions, including our judgment, are gradually becoming dull—the longer we eat in an unnatural manner. People in this condition often find it difficult to understand why they should eat properly. In many cases, their attitude is something like "I have been eating meat for thirty years and am in good health, so why should I stop now?" However, this type of person often has a sudden heart attack or eventually develops cancer.

To further understand the mechanism of sickness, let us consider the difference between *condition* and *constitution*. Since our condition is a result of our day-to-day eating, it is always changing. On the other hand, our constitution changes very slowly, if at all. Our constitution can be thought of as our original condition. In other words, our constitution represents our condition while in the mother's womb, and is determined by our mother's diet. After birth, this becomes our constitution, which continues to be formed until about the age of twenty-four for men and twenty-two for women. This process is accomplished with the appearance of wisdom teeth. In general, degenerative diseases affect the constitution, while adjustments represent changes in condition.

The Seven Levels of Eating

Eating is the most important function in life, since without it, life would not exist. It is the single most important factor in determining whether or not we are harmonious with our environment, and therefore, whether we are healthy or sick. As with sickness, there are seven general levels of eating:

1. Mechanical Eating. An example of this is the way we eat while in the mother's womb, which is without consciousness or desire. However, some people continue to eat this way even after becoming adult. An example is when we come home in the evening and automatically go to the refrigerator for something to eat, often without even washing our hands or taking off our coats. Even dogs or other animals are more conscious of their eating than this. Another example is when we automatically eat at a certain specified time, such as 12 Noon or 6 P.M., even if we aren't hungry.

2. Sensory Eating. This level of eating follows as our senses begin to develop soon after we are born, and is based on our preference for certain tastes, odors, colors and textures. The food industry is presently making huge profits as a result of catering to these desires, since the overwhelming majority of people eat on this level. However, as with the mechanical level, this type of eating will eventually spoil our health.

3. Sentimental or Emotional Eating. Even though we may not want to, when we go out with friends, many of us eat this way in order to be sociable. Candlelight dinners accompanied by music are also examples of sentimental eating. We eat on this level when we visit our relatives' homes and eat what they are eating in order to satisfy them. About 99% of modern people are eating on these first three levels, all of which produce an eventual deterioration of our health.

4. Intellectual Eating. This level of eating is based on nutritional recommendations which are advocated mostly by professional nutritionists and dieticians. At present, this represents the highest popular level of eating in America, and it is more popular among scientists and university professors. For the most part, however, these systems and theories are unworkable. The United States is the richest country in the world, so some people in America may be able to practice these suggestions; yet, even among Americans, many cannot afford to eat this way. As far as other countries are concerned, there are millions of people who cannot afford to buy meat, milk, and other expensive food items on a regular basis. This level of eating is only possible for a small number of people and has no universal value. Besides, rather than being beneficial for human health, many nutritional theories are often harmful.

5. Social Eating. At this level, one realizes that 98 % of the world's people cannot afford to eat according to nutritional theories, and that this type of eating is even too complicated and time-consuming for most of the people who recommend it. For example, it is unlikely that the wives of dieticians or nutritionists actually keep track of vitamins, protein, minerals, etc., when they shop for food. Most probably, they go to the supermarket and buy whatever they want, as do other wives. Although many of these theories sound wonderful, they are usually impractical for most people.

The social level of eating takes place when we start to think in terms of the economics of food. An example is when someone can afford meat, eggs, and milk, but doesn't use many of these items so as to be able to contribute toward helping to feed people who are less fortunate. The concept of social eating developed in relatively recent times, particularly with the advent of socialism and communism, and is more widespread in countries with these forms of government, while the intellectual level is more widespread in democratic countries. The social way of eating is not necessarily the most ideal, however, since the emphasis is more on quantity rather than quality.

6. Ideological Eating. The dietary customs of many religions, such as the dietary teachings of Moses, Jesus, Buddha, Mohammed, and others are examples of this. Unfortunately, since their nature is limited to specific environments where they originally developed, they have all declined. For example, there are few Kosher restaurants in Jewish neighborhoods now, and few Christians eat in a manner similar to Jesus. The same is true in Zen Buddhism. If you visit a Zen monastery, you will discover that the monks are eating white refined rice, sugar, and other processed foods instead of brown rice, vegetables, and other natural foods which were traditionally served.

7. Free Eating. This does not mean chaotic eating, but eating freely in harmony with the order of the universe. For example, if you visit a place such as Israel, Pakistan, or South America, the best thing to do is to study the traditional dietary customs of the people who have been living there for thousands of years. This basic diet can then be modified according to seasonal change and personal need. Free eating means the ability to freely adapt to our surroundings. At this level, we use free will in selecting food according to our freely-chosen purpose, and as a result, health and happiness automatically follow. When properly understood and applied, the macrobiotic way of eating represents this level, since it is based on a flexible adaptation to nature and the universe. At the same time, it also satisfies all of the previous levels of eating.

CHAPTER TWO

The Progressive Development of Sickness

The macrobiotic way of natural healing is not limited to the relief of symptoms. It is equally concerned with educating people toward an understanding and practice of a way of life in harmony with nature and the universe. Health and happiness are the result of living in harmony with nature, while sickness is the consequence of acting, thinking, and living in a manner that is disharmonious. If, through our free will, we choose to disharmonize ourselves with our environment, sickness will occur as the natural process through which balance is again restored. Therefore, the most fundamental way of approaching sickness is to restore ourselves to a condition of harmony with the universe. This is actually the normal human condition, and it can be achieved through the following methods:

1.   Dietary Approach.   Proper eating is the most basic way of establishing harmony with our environment. If our daily food is in accord with our surroundings, our blood, cells, and therefore emotions, thoughts, and consciousness will also be in accord. Harmony is created through the union of opposites: for example, man and woman as well as the union of countless other complemental phenomena in the universe. The union of man and woman is referred to as *sex*, while the union of human beings with the vegetable kingdom is known as *eating*. Proper eating is the essence of natural healing, and without it, sickness can never be definitively cured.

2.   Mental Approach.   Sickness is also an indication that our thinking has grown out of order. Persons with any type of sickness should view the healing process as being one of learning how to adapt and maintain harmony with nature and the universe. This type of education is actually the most important of any that we receive.

The Standard Way of Macrobiotic Eating

The standard macrobiotic way of eating represents a set of general guidelines for dietary practice in a temperate, or four-season climate. This way of eating is the most moderate in terms of yin and yang balance, and will naturally produce a condition of harmonious adaptability to the surrounding environment and result in the development and maintenance of health. However, the majority of people are not eating this way, which means that their diets contain an abundance of foods which are extremely yin or extremely yang or both. Almost every modern degenerative illness, including cancer, heart disease, and multiple sclerosis, results from the habitual excessive intake of foods which are either too yang, too yin, or both.
   This standard diet consists of the following:
   1.   At least 50% of the volume of every meal should be whole cereal grains,

prepared in a variety of cooking methods. Whole cereal grains include brown rice, whole wheat (in the form of bread, chapati, noodles), barley, millet, oats, oatmeal, corn (on the cob, as grits or meal), buckwheat (groats or noodles), rye, etc.

2. Approximately 5% of daily food intake by volume should include soup, preferably seasoned with *miso* or *tamari* (one or two small bowls). The taste should not be too salty. The ingredients should include a variety of vegetables, seaweeds, beans, and grains, and the recipe should often vary.

3. About 20%–30% of each meal may include vegetables. These should be locally grown and in season, or else seasonal vegetables that can be naturally stored. Two-thirds of these should be cooked in various ways, including sautéing, steaming, boiling, and baking; while the remaining third may be eaten raw or as lightly boiled salad.

4. From 10% to 15% of daily intake should include cooked beans and seaweed. Beans for daily use are *azuki* beans, chickpeas, lentils, and black beans. Other beans are for occasional use only. Seaweeds such as *hijiki*, *kombu*, *wakame*, *nori*, dulse, agar-agar, and Irish moss can be prepared with a variety of cooking methods. These dishes should be flavored with a moderate amount of *tamari* soy sauce or sea salt.

5. Beverages should include (1) *bancha* twig tea, roasted; (2) *Mu* tea; (3) dandelion tea; (4) cereal grain tea or coffee; and (5) any traditional tea which is not artificially produced or does not have an aromatic fragrance and stimulant effect.

This comprises the standard macrobiotic way of eating, to which the following supplements may be occasionally added:

1. Once or twice a week, a small volume of white meat fish or shellfish may be eaten. The method of cooking should vary every week, and the volume of fish should always be less than 15% of the meal.

2. A cooked fruit dessert may also be eaten two or three times per week, provided the fruits grow in the local climatic zone and are in season. In a temperate zone, tropical and semi-tropical fruits should be avoided. Fruit juice is not advisable, although it may be used occasionally in hot weather.

3. Roasted seeds or roasted nuts, lightly seasoned with salt or *tamari*, may be enjoyed as a snack or supplement as well as dried fruit and roasted beans.*

The following are additional suggestions for the practice of this standard way of eating:

1. Cooking oil should be of vegetable origin. If you wish to improve your health, limit oil to good quality sesame oil and corn oil in moderate quantity.

2. Salt should be unrefined sea salt. *Tamari* soy sauce and *miso*, prepared in

---

* That a way of eating similar to the above is beneficial for the prevention of disease is being recognized by an increasing number of doctors and nutritionists, as well as by the public at large. For example, in the report entitled *Dietary Goals for the United States* released early in 1977 by the Select Committee on Nutrition and Human Needs of the United States Senate under the chairmanship of Senator George McGovern, Americans were advised to increase their intake of whole grains, beans, and fresh vegetables and fruits, in order to reduce the risk of serious illness. The dietary recommendations contained in this report approach the standard macrobiotic way of eating.

the traditional way, may be used as salty seasoning. In general, food should be moderately or lightly seasoned, and should not have a salty taste.

3. The following condiments are recommended:
   —*Gomasio* (10 to 12 parts roasted sesame seeds to 1 part sea salt, ground together in a small earthenware bowl, or *suribachi*).
   —Roasted kelp (*kombu*) powder or roasted *wakame* powder. (Roast in oven until crisp, then crush in *suribachi*.)
   —*Umeboshi* plums
   —*Tekka*
   —*Tamari* soy sauce (moderate use only)

4. You may eat one, two, or three meals per day, or as much as you want, provided the proportion is correct and chewing is thorough. Each mouthful should be chewed 50 times or more. Avoid eating for approximately three hours before sleeping. For thirst, you may drink a small amount of water, but not iced.

5. Proper cooking is so important that everyone is advised to learn the way of cooking by attending classes or through advice from experienced macrobiotic cooks. Various books and publications on the art of macrobiotic cooking may also be consulted.

In addition, the following practices are recommended for the establishment and maintenance of health and happiness:

1. Let us live happily without being preoccupied about our condition, and let us be active both mentally and physically.

2. Let us be grateful for everything and everyone, and let us offer thanks before and after each meal.

3. Whenever possible, try to retire before midnight and rise early in the morning.

4. Try to avoid wearing synthetic or woolen clothing directly in contact with the body, as well as using excessive metallic accessories on the fingers, wrists, or neck, keeping such ornaments as simple and graceful as possible.

5. If your strength permits, go outdoors often in simple clothing, and, if possible, barefoot. Try to walk on the grass and soil every fine day for up to one half-hour.

6. Try to keep your home in good order, starting from the kitchen, bathroom, bedroom, and living rooms, and including every corner of the house.

7. Initiate and maintain an active correspondence, extending your love and friendship towards parents, brothers and sisters, relatives, teachers, and friends.

8. Avoid taking long baths or showers unless you have been consuming too much salt or animal food.

9. Scrub your whole body with either a hot damp towel or a dry towel until the skin becomes red, every morning or every night before retiring. If that is not possible, at least do your hands and feet, including each finger and toe.

10. Avoid the use of chemically perfumed cosmetics. For care of the teeth, brush with natural preparations or sea salt.

11. If your physical condition allows, try to exercise vigorously on a regular basis, including such activities as scrubbing floors, cleaning windows, washing

clothes, yoga, martial arts, sports, and other forms of systematic exercise.

The Modern Diet

1. Foods Which Are More Yang

Many of the foods being consumed at present on a regular basis are more yang than those included in the standard diet. These products, which many people are eating daily, include:
— Eggs
— Meat (beef, pork, lamb, and others)
— Poultry (chicken, turkey, and others)
— Salt: Salt is often used as a preservative in order to prevent the putrefaction of meat and other animal products. Products like ham, bacon, hot dogs, and others are often preserved in this manner, and salt is often added after they have been cooked. In case salt is not used, chemicals are added to prevent putrefaction. These produce an opposite, or yin, effect. If we consume products such as these on a regular basis, our intake of salt tends to be too large.
— Cheese (more salty varieties)

2. Foods Which Are More Yin

The following products, all of which are being consumed regularly, are more yin than those included in the standard diet:
— Chemicals (additives, sprays, fertilizers, drugs, medications, etc.)
— Sugar
— Chocolate
— Honey, maple syrup, and other simple sugars
— Saccharine and other artificial sweeteners
— Soft drinks and other artificial beverages
— Tropical and semi-tropical fruits such as oranges, grapefruit, benanas, pineapples, mangoes, papayas, etc.
— Vegetables of tropical or semi-tropical origin including potatoes, tomatoes, eggplant, avocados, etc.
— Vegetables which produce an acidic effect such as asparagus, spinach, beets, zucchini squash, green pepper, and others
— Industrially produced, artificial vinegar
— Dairy products which are industrially processed and chemically treated such as milk, butter, cheese (for example, cottage cheese, cream cheese and others), and yoghurt
— Refined flour and grain products
— Spicy condiments and seasonings such as catsup, mustard, pepper, red pepper, and others
— Alcohol
— Commercially produced tea and coffee
— Aromatic teas which have a stimulant effect like mint or peppermint teas.

The present diet of the vast majority of people includes foods from both of these categories. If we regularly eat foods in either of these groups, we are automatically attracted to the foods in the other. Everyone is balancing yin and yang, but in most cases, this balance is maintained intuitively without conscious awareness. However, foods such as those outlined above are very difficult to balance. After 10, 20 or 30 years of eating foods from these categories, your condition will become either excessively yang, excessively yin, or both. In general, a diet of this type results in a very chaotic state of chronic imbalance.

In general, the foods included in both categories produce an acidic condition in the bloodstream. Among the foods included as a part of the standard diet, which are all more centrally balanced, some create a mildly acid condition while others produce milk alkaline. On the whole, a diet of this type will cause a weak alkaline condition to be maintained in the bloodstream.

A Nutritional Approach to Cancer

When foods which are at the extremes of yin or yang comprise the mainstay of our diet for any length of time, our physiological condition becomes imbalanced. Since the body at all times seeks balance with the surrounding environment, the normal process is for this excess to be eliminated, or stored when it exceeds the body's capacity for elimination. Let us consider the progressive stages in this process, particularly in their relation to the eventual development of cancer.

1. Normal Elimination

Normal elimination occurs through the processes of urination, bowel movement, respiration (exhaling CO_2), and perspiration, in which excessive chemical compounds are broken down into simple compounds, and ultimately, into carbon dioxide and water, which are then discharged. Discharge also occurs through physical, mental, and emotional activity. Mental discharge occurs in the form of wave vibrations, while emotions such as anger indicate that a great amount of excess is being discharged.

Women have several additional means through which excess is naturally discharged. These include menstruation, childbirth, and lactation. Women have a distinct advantage over men in more efficiently discharging excess and thereby maintaining a cleaner or purer condition. To compensate for this, men usually go out into society and discharge through additional physical, mental, and social activities. All of these processes take place continually throughout life. If we take in a moderate amount of excess, they will proceed smoothly. However, if the quantity of excess is large, these natural processes are not capable of discharging it, and at this time, various abnormal processes begin.

2. Abnormal Discharge

These processes occur from time to time and include abnormal symptoms such as

(1) fever, (2) coughing, (3) diarrhea, (4) frequent urination, (5) abnormal sweating, and (6) abnormal motions such as shivering, shaking legs, etc. This type of discharge can also occur through abnormal thoughts and emotions. Discharges of this type represent various types of adjustment sicknesses, and their frequency depends on the quantity of unnecessary excess that is taken in. In many cases, however, the continuous intake of excess exceeds even these channels of discharge. This often leads to the elimination of excess through the skin.

3. The Development of Skin Disease

A. General Skin Disorders. The most common causes of skin disorders are animal foods—e.g., meat, eggs, dairy, and fish—followed by sugar, fruit juice, oil, and other yin products. When approaching skin diseases, we should not try to suppress this discharge; rather, we should encourage it to come out while at the same time eliminating the cause of the problem. A person with skin disease should begin the standard diet and avoid the following foods until the condition clears up: (1) all animal products; (2) buckwheat; (3) various types of extremely yin foods such as fruit and sweets; (4) all raw foods including even a small quantity of salad; (5) "quick" pickles which are aged less than two months; and (6) flour products.

It is very important for a person with any type of skin disease to eat cooked foods only. For example, several years ago I met a woman who had been suffering from skin disease for over twenty years. Her condition had prevented her from getting married and even from finding a job. The cause of her problem had been her intake of sugar, and after two weeks of proper eating, her condition had improved about 50%. When I saw her again after another two weeks, she had improved only slightly. This improvement was not as good as it could have been, and this was the result of her having eaten a small salad every day. After she stopped her intake of salad, the problem cleared up completely.

The following external treatments are also helpful in relieving skin diseases by speeding up the process of discharge:

1. *Compress Made from Dried Leaves and Grated Ginger:* Boil dried leaves, using the method described in the chapter, *The Reproductive System* in the section on the treatment of female disorders. Grate fresh ginger root and wrap in cheesecloth. Turn off the flame, and place this "ginger sack" (which should contain a lump of grated ginger about the size of a golf ball) in the water. Then, dip a towel into the water, squeeze, and apply to the affected area.

2. *Rice Bran* Nuka *Skin Wash:* Wrap *nuka* in cheesecloth. Place in hot water and shake. The *nuka* will melt and the water will begin to turn yellow. Then, wash the affected area with a towel or cloth that has been dipped in this water.

3. *Wood Ash Skin Wash:* Place ashes that are left over after burning wood in a fireplace into hot water and stir very well. Let sit until the ashes settle to the bottom, and then use the water to wash the skin. Pat dry with a towel.

4. Daikon *Application:* In cases where a person with skin disease suffers itching, rub a piece of cut fresh *daikon* directly onto the affected area. If you don't have *daikon*, use a scallion or onion.

5. *Sesame Oil Application:* Sesame oil can be applied directly to the affected area in cases where the skin becomes ruptured.

Persons with skin diseases should avoid using blankets which are made of wool or synthetic fibers, and ideally these should be cotton. Clothing should also be made of cotton or other natural vegetable fibers. This is especially important in the case of underclothing. Rice bran which is wrapped in cheesecloth or natural vegetable-quality soaps should be used instead of chemical soaps or shampoos.

These diseases usually appear when the intestines and kidneys become incapable of efficiently discharging toxins. The intestines and kidneys can be strengthened through the use of hot applications along with proper eating. The most effective of these is the ginger compress, which should be repeatedly applied directly to these organs. A roasted salt application may be used in place of the ginger compress.

B. Skin Cancer. Skin cancers are more serious forms of skin disease. Persons with these diseases should stop eating all foods which are extremely yang or extremely yin, and should begin the standard macrobiotic way of eating. Within the range of macrobiotic foods, fish, fruit, salad, and nuts should be avoided, although seeds may be eaten on occasion. Thorough chewing is essential to restore the quality of the blood. For any type of cancer, each mouthful must be chewed at least 100, and preferably 200 times. Skin cancers are relatively easy to relieve with this approach, and success can be expected in practically every case. Modern medicine will often treat skin cancer with radiation, chemotherapy, or by surgical removal. These symptomatic approaches reveal an incomplete understanding of the cause of this disease, or of the possibility of eliminating it from the inside by removing the cause. Although these approaches may eliminate the external symptoms, the disease will reappear if the patient does not change his internal quality.

Skin diseases are usually not very serious, since in most cases, the discharge of toxins permits the internal organs and tissues to continue functioning smoothly. However, if our eating continues to be excessive, the body will start to accumulate this excess.

4. Accumulation

At this stage, the volume of excess exceeds the body's capacity for discharging it, and it begins to accumulate. However, this excess tends to be deposited toward the periphery of the body, particularly in regions that come in contact with the outside. Let us consider each of these in some detail.

A. The Sinuses. The sinuses are the most common site for the accumulation of excess. Mucus will often accumulate in this area so that it may be discharged through the nose and from the eyes. Often, when dust or pollen enters the nostrils, the mucous membranes react in an effort to push as much excess as possible toward the outside. Reactions such as this are known as hay fever or allergies, and are nothing but discharge mechanisms.

To diagnose sinus trouble, refer to the pressure-points indicated in the section on pressure-point diagnosis. If these points are painful when pressed, there are mucus deposits in the sinuses. Moxa can be applied to these points to help relieve this condition. If moxa is not available, a lighted cigarette can be used as a substitute, preferably a brand in which the tobacco is tightly packed. To apply cigarette moxa, refer to the technique outlined in the section on pressure-point diagnosis. By applying moxa to these points twice each day for several days, the deposited mucus will begin to loosen.

Another external application that is helpful in relieving sinus congestion is a *lotus root plaster*. This method can help to dissolve mucus which has taken years to accumulate. Before applying this plaster, apply a hot water or ginger compress to the sinus region. These compresses can be discontinued when the skin turns red, and should be followed immediately with the lotus root plaster.

To make the plaster, grate a piece of fresh lotus root (which is available in most oriental or natural food stores) without peeling it. If the grated pulp is thin and watery, thicken with about 10%–15% white flour. The grated pulp should have a pasty consistency. Add about 5% grated ginger and mix well. This mixture should then be applied directly to the skin to a thickness of about 2/3 of an inch, covering the entire region of the sinuses, especially the forehead and around the nose, and can be held in place with a cotton bandage that is wrapped around the head. Apply this plaster right before going to bed, and leave it on until the following morning, at which time the lotus root can simply be washed off. This procedure should be repeated over several consecutive evenings, after which a large quantity of mucus will often start to be discharged. This discharge may include deposits of mucus which have been in the sinuses for years, as well as calcified stones, which are often discharged through sneezing.

B. The Inner Ear. The accumulation of mucus and fat in the inner ear can lead to frequent pain, impaired hearing, and even deafness. In America, more than 12 million people are deaf, and this number is steadily increasing. If this continues for another 25 years, 50% of the American population may become deaf. The mechanism of hearing troubles is discussed in our chapter, *The Face and Head*, along with several methods for treating these disorders.

To diagnose problems in the inner ear, use the points located in the indented region directly below each ear which are mentioned in the section on pressure-point diagnosis. Pain indicates that mucus is beginning to accumulate. Cigarette moxa can be applied to these points to help relieve this condition. Another helpful treatment is to slowly circle each ear with a lighted cigarette which is held about 1/4 inch from the skin. After several circuits, the person's body will begin to feel warm, particularly in the area of the kidneys, since these organs correspond to the ears.

C. The Lungs. Excess in various forms will often accumulate in the lungs. Aside from the obvious symptoms of coughing and chest congestion, this condition can be diagnosed by pushing with your finger in the area under the vocal cords in the center of the throat. If this is painful, the lungs have begun to accumulate mucus which has the possibility of developing into some type of cyst or into cancer.

To help relieve this condition, apply a ginger compress to the area of the lungs, using either the front or the back of the body. The compress can be applied once each day for 10 days or two weeks, and it will help to loosen stagnation in this area by stimulating the circulation of blood. The mechanism whereby accumulated mucus develops into more serious problems such as lung cancer is discussed in our chapter, *The Respiratory System.*

D.   The Breasts.   The accumulation of excess in this area often results in a hardening of the breasts, as well as in the formation of cysts. Excess usually accumulates in the breasts in the form of mucus and deposits of fatty acid, both of which take the form of a yin, sticky or heavy liquid. These deposits develop into cysts in the same way that water freezes into ice, and this occurs when foods like ice cream, sugar, orange juice, soft drinks, and other cold beverages are consumed on a regular basis. All of these produce a cooling effect which causes these stored deposits to crystallize.

   Aside from proper eating, the primary method of relieving this condition is to literally "melt away" these hard deposits. These methods are discussed later in this chapter.

E.   The Intestines.   In many cases, excess will begin accumulating in the lower part of the body in the form of mucus and fat deposits which coat the intestinal wall. This will often cause the intestines to expand, resulting in a bulging abdomen. A large number of people in the United States have this problem, and Americans have acquired an international notariety for this. Young people in America are often very stylish and attractive. However, after the age of 30, and particularly between the ages of 35 and 40, a large number of Americans lose their youthful appearance and become overweight and unattractive.

F.   The Kidneys.   The kidneys are a frequent site of mucus and fatty-acid accumulation, since they are connected to the outside through the bladder and urinary tract. Problems arise when these elements cannot pass through the fine network of cells in the interior of these organs. In this condition, the kidneys often accumulate water and become chronically swollen. Since the process of elimination is hampered, fluid which cannot be discharged is often deposited in the legs, producing periodic swelling and weakness. At the same time, a person with this condition often perspires excessively.

   If someone with this condition consumes a large quantity of foods which produce a chilling effect, such as those mentioned in our discussion of breast cysts, the deposited fat and mucus will often crystallize into stones. In order to dissolve these stones, we need to eat foods which have the effect of dissolving or melting these deposits. Vegetables like *daikon* radish, ginger, and turnips are very effective for this, and can be cooked in soups, with other vegetables, or, in the case of *daikon*, grated and eaten raw. These should be included within the standard macrobiotic way of eating.

   A hot ginger compress applied daily will cause most kidney stones to begin melting and shrinking in size, while some may even split into several pieces. As their size becomes smaller, they will begin to pass through the ureter into the bladder, where they are discharged during urination. In some cases, the stones or stone fragments are too large to pass smoothly through the ureter. This often results in a very sharp pain that is often mistaken for an appendicitis attack. However, appendicitis is accompanied by a fever, whereas the discharge of a kidney stone is not. If the pain from this discharge becomes intolerable, and we go to a hospital, the stone will most likely be surgically removed. However, this is unnecessary, since the pain can be relieved by applying a ginger compress to the area and by drinking plenty of hot *bancha* tea. This will cause the ureter to dilate and allow the stone to pass through. Salt or salty foods should not be eaten at this time, since they will cause the ureter to contract, thereby increasing the pain.

For additional relief, cigarette moxa can be applied to the kidney point at the bottom of the foot as well as to the point above the ankle on the inside of the leg known as *San-In-Ko*. The location of these points can be found in the chapter. *The Way of Diagnosis*, in the section *Pressure-Point Diagnosis*.

Kidney stones can be eliminated very easily through the proper application of the standard diet, combined with the additional treatments mentioned above.

G. The Sexual Organs.   In men, the prostate gland is a frequent site of accumulation. As a result, it often becomes enlarged, and hard fat deposits or cysts often form within and around it. This is one of the principal causes of impotency. The standard macrobiotic way of eating will relieve this condition, along with regular ginger compresses which can be applied to the area of the bladder. For the development of sexual ability, men should be careful not to overeat.

Since the female sexual organs are connected to the outside, excess will often accumulate there. This often leads to the formation of ovarian cysts, as well as to blockage of the Fallopian tubes. In many cases, mucus or fat in the ovaries or Fallopian tubes will prevent the passage of the egg and sperm, resulting in an inability to conceive. The treatment for this condition, as well as for the related problem of vaginal discharges, is discussed in our chapter, *The Reproductive System*.

All of these forms of accumulation can be eliminated through the methods that we have just discussed. However, if we ignore these conditions, or if we try some type of symptomatic measure such as having an operation, taking medication, or merely quitting smoking, without changing our diet, we inevitably proceed to the next stage.

5. Storage

In this stage, excess in various forms is stored within and around the internal organs, resulting in their improper functioning. In the case of the circulatory system, excess often accumulates around and inside the heart, as well as within the heart tissues. Accumulation may also occur both in and around the arteries. These fatty deposits reduce the heart's ability to function properly and hampers the smooth passage of blood through the arteries. The end result is often a heart attack. The major causes of this problem are foods which contain large amounts of hard, saturated fat. Many nutritionists and doctors are now aware of the relationship between the intake of saturated fats, cholesterol, and cardiovascular disease, but often overlook the effect of sugar and dairy products, both of which contribute greatly to the development of these illnesses.

Within the body, the proteins, carbohydrates, and fats that we consume often change into each other, depending on the amount of each consumed as well as the body's needs at a particular time. If we consume more of these than we need, this excess is normally discharged. However, the quantity of excess often exceeds the body's capacity to discharge it. When this happens, the excess is stored in the liver in the form of carbohydrate, in the muscles in the form of protein, or throughout the body in the form of fatty acids. (See Fig. 1.)

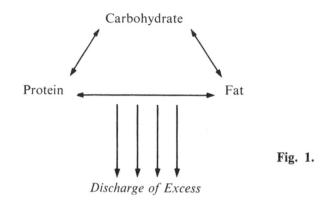

Fig. 1.

Discharge of Excess

In the heart, accumulated fatty deposits are usually not distributed evenly. For example, one side of the heart will often contain more than the other, and this imbalance will cause the rhythm of the heart to become irregular. If the storage of excess continues in this manner, breathing becomes difficult, and, since the lungs are usually accumulating mucus while the heart accumulates fatty deposits, the ability of the lungs to absorb oxygen and discharge carbon dioxide is substantially impeded.

The tip of the nose reflects the condition of the circulatory system and in particular the heart, with the left and right sides of the nose corresponding to the left and right sides of the heart respectively. If the left side of the nose is harder than the right, because of deposits of hard fat, this indicates that fatty deposits are also greater in the left side of the heart. The resulting improper coordination of the heartbeat often produces a heart murmur.

The whole face is a reflection of the condition of the heart. If the face has a reddish color or a swollen appearance, this indicates that the heart is also swollen and expanded. A pale face means that the circulation within the heart is weak, and that the heart tissues are not receiving enough blood. An oily or greasy complexion means that the heart is coated with fatty deposits. The location of pimples and other facial blemishes indicates the region of the heart in which fatty deposits are most prevalent. For example, pimples on the lower left side of the face indicate that the lower left side of the heart contains a high concentration of fatty deposits. (See Fig. 2.)

6. Chronic Blood-Lymph Degeneration Leading to Cancer

If the bloodstream is filled with fat and mucus, excess will begin to accumulate in the organs. Since the lungs and kidneys are usually affected first, their functions of filtering and cleansing the blood become less efficient. This situation leads to further deterioration of the blood quality and also affects the lymphatic system. Operations

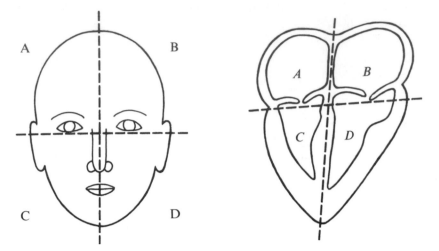

Fig. 2. *The condition of the heart can be seen in the entire face. The correspondences between the two are illustrated in the above diagram.*

such as tonsilectomies also contribute to the deterioration of the lymphatic system, since they reduce the ability of this system to cleanse itself. Such operations eventually lead to frequent swelling and lymph gland inflammation, producing a chronic deterioration of the quality of the blood, particularly the red blood cells. When the red blood cells then begin to lose their capacity to change into normal body cells, they start to create the degenerate type of cell that is known as cancerous.

Poorly functioning intestines can also contribute to the degeneration of blood quality, since blood cells and plasma originate largely in the small intestine. In many cases, the villi of the small intestine are coated with fat and mucus, and the condition in the intestines is often acidic. Naturally, healthy blood will not be created in this type of environment.

A. Nutrition and the Cause of Cancer. Cancer develops from chronic degeneration of the blood and lymph fluid. Once we realize that cancer is the result of a general body-wide deterioration, we can better appreciate the body's attempt to concentrate the cancerous cells in a particular location to prevent the organism as a whole from being poisoned. The location of this concentration depends upon which type of food is primarily responsible for the formation of the cancerous cells. (See Fig. 3.)

△ YANG ORGANS *more solid and compact*	▽ YIN ORGANS *more hollow and expanded*
Lungs	Large Intestine
Heart	Small Intestine
Kidney	Bladder
Spleen/Pancreas	Stomach
Liver	Gall Bladder

Fig. 3.

In general, there are two types of cancer, which we can classify according to cause. The first results from excess yang foods such as eggs, meat, fish, and some types of dairy food. The second is caused by excessive intake of yin, such as soft drinks, sugar, milk, citrus, stimulants, chemicals, refined flour and grain products, and spices. In general, if the cancer appears in the more deep parts of the body, or if it involves the more yang, compacted organs (listed above), it is caused by the over-consumption of yang foods. Yin-caused cancers usually develop at the periphery of the body, or in the more yin, hollow organs. However, this classification is not absolute. Although cancer arises as the result of a predominance of one factor, the opposite factor is also involved, even though to a lesser degree. For example, cancers which result from the overconsumption of yang foods also require an intake of yin, since this provides the stimulus for tumor growth.

Thus, cancer was unknown among the Eskimos until sugar and other products of civilization were introduced. The inclusion of these extremely yin items provided the necessary stimulus for their normally very yang diet to lead to the formation of a variety of cancers.

Also, regions within each organ have either a more yin or more yang nature. For example, the stomach can be divided into the more expanded region, which secretes strong acid, and the more compact pylorus, which secretes a much weaker acid. The body portion of the stomach is more yin, while the pylorus is more yang, as is the duodenum. Although on the whole the stomach is a yin organ, cancers which appear in the more expanded parts are more yin, resulting from the intake of foods such as sugar, monosodium glutamate (MSG), white refined rice and flour, and other yin products; while those which develop in the more yang pylorus or duodenum result from the overconsumption of meat, eggs, fish, and other more yang products. Since these more yin foods are consumed widely in Japan, the people in that nation have a very high incidence of stomach cancer, while other types of cancer, such as those resulting from the intake of saturated fat, are more predominant in America. (See Fig. 4.)

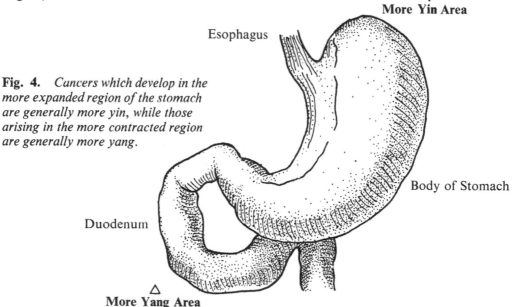

▽
More Yin Area

Esophagus

Fig. 4. *Cancers which develop in the more expanded region of the stomach are generally more yin, while those arising in the more contracted region are generally more yang.*

Body of Stomach

Duodenum

△
More Yang Area

The ascending colon is the most yin part of the large intestine. The rectum, being more tight and narrow, is the most yang part, while the transverse and descending portions of the colon have both yin and yang characteristics. If cancer arises in the yin, ascending colon, it is caused by the overconsumption of yin foods such as honey, white refined flour, milk, fruit juice, sugar, saccharine, and others. Conversely, cancer of the rectum is caused more by yang foods such as eggs, meat, and some types of cheese, although yin foods are also involved. Cancer of the transverse or descending colon results from a combination of excessively yin and excessively yang foods. (See Fig. 5.)

Cancer of the liver, spleen, and pancreas results from the overconsumption of yang foods. Tumors or cancers which arise in the compact brain also have as their base the consumption of yang foods. Brain tumors are relatively easy to relieve through proper eating since (1) tumors in this very compact area tend to grow very slowly, and (2) the abundance of blood supply to the brain means that a change in blood quality will quickly affect the condition of the brain.

Cancer of the small intestine is generally yin, but it also involves a contributing factor from various yang foods. Uterine cancer arises from the combination of both extremes, as does breast cancer. The saturated fats contained in meat, eggs, and dairy products combine with the effects of sugar and other yin products to produce these conditions. Prostate cancer is generally the result of too many yin foods, but, among yin cancers, it is a more yang variety, similar in degree to cancer of the descending colon. Skin cancer results from the excessive intake of yin foods like dairy, sugar, and honey, combined with various types of yang animal foods. Skin conditions like psoriasis and eczema may be considered as pre-cancerous conditions, as are white or brown patches which appear on the skin.

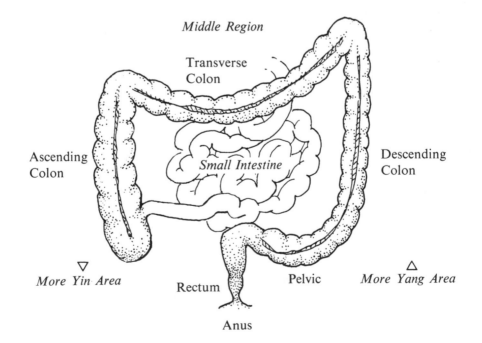

Fig. 5. *Large Intestine (Colon).*

B. A Dietary Approach to Cancer. When studying a case of cancer, one should first try to determine whether the person's overall condition is more yin or more yang. On the whole, suggestions should be directed primarily toward restoring the individual's excessively yin or yang condition to one that is less extreme. Once a more neutral or balanced condition has been stabilized, the person's body no longer accumulates and concentrates toxins in the form of cancer. If one keeps this wholistic view in mind, one can avoid being caught in an endless maze of symptoms.

Dietary recommendations must vary depending on whether the cancer is of a more yin or yang origin. That can usually be determined by noting the location of the cancer and the person's general condition and eating habits. In the case of yang cancers, we should recommend the standard macrobiotic way of eating, modifying it slightly so as to accentuate more yin factors. The reverse is true in the case of yin cancers. However, extremes of either yin or yang must be avoided, since these are what initially caused the cancer to develop. When uncertain whether the cancer is from a yin or a yang origin, one can safely recommend the balanced, central diet. The variations in the standard diet according to the type of cancer are indicated in Fig. 6.

Since cancer is a symptom of excess, a person with this disease must be careful not to overeat. Two very important practices can be followed in order to prevent this. First, each mouthful of food should be chewed thoroughly—at least 100, and preferably 200 times. A person with cancer may eat as much food as he or she wants, provided it is well-chewed and thoroughly mixed with saliva. The second caution is not to eat for at least three hours before going to bed, since food eaten at this time becomes surplus which will serve to accelerate the growth of the cancer. Regarding liquid intake, the individual should not drink unless thirsty. Also, a normal amount of physical activity should be maintained if possible.

Of course, in order to make a responsible decision, a person with cancer must understand that he or she was responsible for the development of the disease through his or her diet, manner of thinking, and way of life. However, once the decision has been made to change, the person should forget about the sickness and live as happily, actively, and normally as possible. Cancer patients are often depressed: therefore, once a person with cancer begins to eat a healthy diet, he or she should be encouraged not to worry but to maintain an optimistic attitude.

A more complex situation occurs if someone has received chemotherapy, cobalt radiation, or has had surgery. However, there is still a good possibility of recovery as long as the patient has normal appetite, good vitality, and the will to live. In a situation like this, it is vital for both the patient and the members of his or her family to understand the importance of properly implementing the dietary recommendations. Ideally, they should spend several days or weeks learning how to cook properly, and should seek qualified advice on the correct manner of eating. The patient should also reflect on the various aspects of his life which led to development of cancer.

Cases that are even more serious—so-called terminal cases—require additional attention. In these situations, the cancer may be rapidly spreading and the patient may be in great pain, and his or her appetite may be diminishing. Such cases require the use of external applications along with the proper way of eating. Food should be cooked to the normal texture and consistency, provided the patient is able to chew

▽ CANCER FROM YIN CAUSE	FOOD	△ CANCER FROM YANG CAUSE
50%–70%	GRAINS	40%–50% (avoid buckwheat)
1 : 8–1 : 10	*GOMASIO*	1 : 10–1 : 14
Thick taste	SOUP (*miso*, *tamari* broth)	Light taste
Longer cooking (10–14 minutes) slightly salty taste	VEGETABLES	Shorter cooking (2–10 minutes) almost no salt taste
Azuki, chickpea lentil	BEANS	Almost any bean
Longer cooking, thicker taste (*hijiki*)	SEAWEED	Quicker cooking, lighter taste (*wakame*, *nori*, dulse)
Strong *bancha* tea or grain coffee, *Mu* tea	BEVERAGE	Light *bancha* tea or grain coffee, no *Mu* tea
None or occasional, preferably boiled for 3 minutes.	SALAD	Up to 10% of meal
No fruit	FRUIT	If crave, may use occasionally dried or cooked fruit or small quantity of fresh local fruits; no fruit juice.
Sesame only, as little as possible. Apply with brush to prevent burning. No raw oil.	OIL	Sesame or corn for cooking, small amount for sautéing. No raw oil.
If crave, an occasional small quantity of white meat fish or shellfish. However, it is better to avoid.	FISH (seafood)	Avoid completely
Occasional seeds. Nuts should be avoided.	NUTS AND SEEDS	Occasional seeds. Nuts should be avoided.

Fig. 6.

and swallow. If the patient has difficulty in eating food prepared in this manner, it is advisable to mash the food after it has been cooked. It may also be necessary to cook the food with more water than usual, in order for it to have a softer, more creamy consistency. Grains, vegetables, beans, and other foods can be cooked in this manner and then mashed by hand in a *suribachi*. A blender should not be used in for this purpose.

The most important external applications are the ginger compress, taro potato plaster, and buckwheat plaster. The methods for preparing these are outlined in the appendix on external applications. However, let us briefly consider their proper use in cases of cancer.

1. Ginger Compress. The ginger compress should be prepared in the usual manner. However, we should apply it only for a short time to activate the circulation in the affected area, and it should be followed immediately by a taro potato plaster. If we apply a hot ginger compress repeatedly over an extended period, it may accelerate the growth of the cancer, particularly if it is of a yin variety. The ginger compress should be considered only as preparation for the taro plaster, and not as an independent treatment. Apply it for several minutes only.

2. Taro Potato (Albi) Plaster. Taro potato can be obtained from Chinese or Armenian groceries or from a natural foods store. The skin of this vegetable is brown and covered with "hair." The taro potato is grown in Hawaii as well as in the Orient. Smaller taro potatoes are the most effective for use in this plaster.

To prepare the plaster, peel off the skin and grate the white part on a flat grater. Mix the grated potato, which should be in the form of a sticky white pulp, with about 5% grated ginger root, and spread the mixture on a piece of linen to a thickness of about 1/2 inch. The plaster should then be applied to the cancerous area so that the grated mixture comes in direct contact with the skin. (See Fig. 7.)

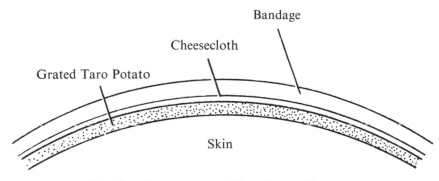

Fig. 7. *Cross-section of Taro Patato Plaster.*

The cool taro application should be put in place immediately following the ginger compress. The taro application can be held in place with a bandage, and should be left on for about four hours, after which its effectiveness decreases. A fresh application should be put on every four hours. If the patient feels chilly because of the coolness of the taro plaster, the hot ginger compress which is applied for five minutes while you are changing plasters will help to relieve this. If a chill persists, roast sea salt in a skillet, wrap it in a towel, and place it on top of the plaster. Be careful not to let the patient become too hot from this salt application.

The taro plaster has the effect of drawing cancerous toxins out of the body, and is particularly effective in removing carbon and other minerals which are contained in tumors. If, when the plaster is removed, the light-colored mixture has become dark or brown, or if the skin where the plaster was applied also takes on a similar color, this change indicates that excessive carbon and other elements are being discharged through the skin. This treatment will gradually decrease the size of the tumor.

Taro potato can usually be obtained in most of the major cities in the United States and Canada. However, if you live in an area where it is not available, a preparation using regular potato can be substituted. Although regular potato is not as effective as taro, it will still produce a beneficial result. Mix 50%–60% grated potato with 40%–50% green leafy vegetables, which should also be grated, by crushing them together in a *suribachi*. Apply this mixture in the same way you would a taro plaster.

3. Buckwheat Plaster. A buckwheat plaster should be applied in cases where a patient develops a swollen abdomen due to the retention of fluid. If this fluid is surgically removed, a patient may temporarily feel better, but after several days, may suddenly become much worse. Obviously, we should try to avoid such a drastic procedure.

To prepare a buckwheat plaster, mix buckwheat flour with warm water and knead it into a dough-like mixture that should be somewhat stiff and not too watery. Apply this to the abdomen to a thickness of about one inch, so that the entire swollen area is covered; hold the plaster in place with a bandage or a piece of cotton linen. This plaster can be applied anywhere on the body. For example, in cases where a breast has been removed, the surrounding lymph nodes, the neck, or in some cases, the arm, often become swollen after several months. To relieve this condition, apply ginger compresses to the swollen area for about five minutes, followed by a buckwheat plaster. The buckwheat plaster should be replaced every four hours. After removing the plaster, you may notice that fluid is starting to come out through the skin, or that the swelling is starting to go down. A buckwheat plaster will usually eliminate the swelling after only several applications, or at most after two or three days.

Most cancers can be dealt with successfully without the use of external treatments. It is only the 20%–30% that are considered terminal or that have been complicated by previous treatment that require these applications. This macrobiotic dietary approach can also be combined with these external applications for the relief of a variety of non-cancerous tumors and cysts including brain tumors, fibroid tumors, ovarian cysts, breast cysts, and others.

The following factors should be considered when judging whether a difficult case of cancer will have a successful outcome:
1. The strength of the person's native constitution.
2. Whether the person has had any previous operations or treatments. Tonsillectomies, appendectomies, and other operations weaken the person's ability to resist and overcome illness, as does the previous use of drugs or medications.
3. Whether the person and his immediate family are capable of self-reflection —in other words, whether they have a spirit of thankfulness and appreciation, not only to the people helping them but also towards life in general, including the marvelous natural defense mechanism of the body.

Without the close cooperation and support of the patient's immediate family, a successful outcome is doubtful. The patient's immediate family should clearly understand the situation and should begin to eat in a similar manner, while extending their love and support to the patient in any possible way.

Due to a small, but steadily increasing, number of cases which seem to indicate that, when the above factors are present, cancer can be relieved through macrobiotic dietary practice, the East West Foundation initiated a conference on the Nutritional Approach to Cancer in 1977. Presented once each year since then, these cancer conferences have been attended by a number of representatives of the medical community, along with international representatives of the macrobiotic community and a number of persons who have experienced what seem to be the relief of a variety of cancers through macrobiotics. The proceedings of these conferences, including case histories and related documentation, are contained in the report, *Cancer and Diet*, available for $4.95 from the East West Foundation, 240 Washington Street, Bookline, MA 02146.

CHAPTER THREE

The Way of Diagnosis

The art of diagnosis forms an integral part of the way of natural healing. Without a clear understanding of the nature of a particular problem, it is difficult, if not impossible, to make the proper recommendations to relieve or solve it. In this chapter, we will outline sixteen different methods of diagnosis, all of which are derived from the understanding of the order of the universe, or natural law. This understanding formed the basis of traditional oriental medicine, and several of these methods have been used for thousands of years in the Far East.

1. Diagnosis from the View of the Total Environment

This type of diagnosis is based on the understanding of our relationship to our large surrounding environment, both in terms of space and in time. This includes the heavenly environment, or *Ten-Sō*, the earthly environment, or *Chi-Sō*, and the environment of time, or *Ji-Sō*. *Sō* can be translated as "phenomena" or "phenomenal appearance." Among these 16 methods of diagnosis, the first six are different forms of *Sō*, while the remainings are varieties of *Shin*, which means "individual symptoms."

A. Ten-Sō: (天相) Heavenly Phenomena. *Ten-Sō* is based on the influence of the different types of celestial motion that affect human life, particularly the motions of the sun, moon, and major constellations. For example, a woman's menstrual cycle varies according to the lunar cycle. This cycle also affects our psychological and emotional condition in general. We are usually more excitable during the full moon, whereas during the new moon we tend to become more quiet. Also, certain sicknesses become more acute during the full moon, while others become active during the new moon. The lunar cycle also influences tides, which produce changes in the atmosphere, which in turn influence the body.

An example of this is asthma, which generally results from the overconsumption of liquid. People with this condition often experience attacks during humid weather. Disorders like headaches, diarrhea, and fevers are also greatly influenced by atmospheric conditions. In treating these problems, we must consider such factors as the position of the sun, the condition of the atmosphere, the phase of the moon, as well as what major constellation is facing the earth at the time of treatment.

B. Chi-Sō: (地相) Earthly Conditions. *Chi-Sō* means our environment on earth. Where we live has a powerful influence on our condition. The mountains, the plains, the seashore, the desert, the fertile valley, the forest, the lake, each affects us in a different way. For example, I recently met a young couple in Amsterdam who were not happy even though they had been eating macrobiotically for several years. The young wife was urinating too frequently, suffered from periodic headaches, and a swollen face, even though she was drinking very little liquid. Thinking that salt was responsible, she had tried avoiding it, but her problem did not improve, although her overall condition had become much better. Her problem was caused by living in a houseboat. Even though she hadn't been drinking excessively, she was constantly breathing in very humid air from the canal on which she was living, and this was the cause of her symptoms.

C. Ji-Sō: (時相) Time.   (See Fig. 8.) Our condition is being constantly influenced by such things as the changing seasons and the cycles of day and night. *Ji-Sō* is the study of the way in which these cycles affect us. As an example, let us consider the problem of polio. Polio is a yin condition, and is caused by the excessive consumption of foods like fruit juice, ice cream, and sugar. When these are eaten excessively, the more yang areas of the body, such as the legs, become weak. Polio is prevalent in the southern United States, where people tend to consume more yin foods than in the North. The consumption of these items tends to be greater during the hot summer months, but during this time, the intense heat somewhat counteracts their effects. After the peak of summer, the weather becomes cooler, and the yin that was consumed during the summer, or that is still being consumed, starts to become excessive, resulting in an overly-yin condition. As a result, polio tends to develop during the late summer and early autumn.

Bedwetting offers a good example of the influence of the 24-hour cycle of day and night. Some children wet their beds soon after going to sleep, while others release urine later in the evening or towards morning. Although the symptom appears to be the same, each has a different cause, depending upon the condition of the bladder.

In some cases, bedwetting occurs when the bladder is contracted and tightly closed, and therefore cannot hold much water; while in others, it results from a loose, expanded bladder which is also unable to hold urine. During which time of night would the bladder be more likely to contract? This would more likely occur later in the evening or towards morning when the atmosphere is darker and colder, or more yin. In the early evening, the atmosphere is not so cold, and the opposite condition, relaxation, would more likely occur. If bedwetting takes place soon after a child goes to bed, the cause is too much yin, including water, fruit juice, spices, various types of sugar, soft drinks, coffee, and similar foods. In the case of an overly-constricted bladder, the cause is too many yang foods like salt, eggs, meat, and fish. For an overly-yang bladder, we should recommend foods which create relaxation. However, we should not advise extremely yin foods like sugar, since these would cause the child's overall condition to deteriorate. Good-quality yin in the form of baked apples, hot apple cider, or any type of cooked, locally-grown, seasonal fruit will help this condition. We should approach an overly-expanded bladder in the opposite way, advising the person to avoid fruits, sugar, and other yin foods, while minimizing the intake of liquid, and including a bit more salt.

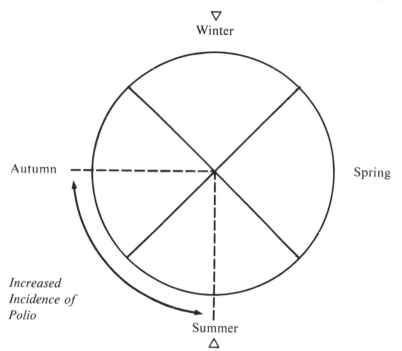

Fig. 8. *Ji-Sō depicts the influence of the seasonal cycle on our physical, emotional and psychological condition. The above diagram illustrates the influence of the seasons on the incidence of polio. Polio occurs more often in the late summer and early autumn. This is due to the accumulated effects of extremely yin foods such as ice cream, soft drinks, and others which tend to be consumed in greater quantities during the hot summer months.*

2. Diagnosis from the View of the Immediate Environment

This method is based on understanding the condition of our direct environment, including factors such as where we live—for example, in the city or country; the type of family that we have; and the nature of our relationships with others. For instance, suppose that a person wishes to change his way of eating, but his wife feels that this is nonsense and continues to serve meat and ice cream. Obviously, it will be difficult for him to eat properly, and as a result, his condition will probably worsen.

As another example, suppose an entire family decides to change their way of eating in order to help a sick member, but that from time to time one of the grandmothers offers the patient honey and fruit. This may prevent the patient from improving his condition. In order for a person to get better, his entire family should extend their full support and cooperation. With this type of encouragement, possibly as many as 98% of all sicknesses can be cured, including many which are considered terminal. On the other hand, it is very difficult to relieve sickness without the full cooperation of the sick person's family.

Another aspect of this type of diagnosis involves seeing the condition of a person's house. For example, a messy, chaotic, or disorderly home is nothing but a reflection of an individual's physical and psychological condition. Also, the condition of a woman's pocketbook reveals much about her health. A disorderly handbag is a reflection of a disorderly condition. The most important room in any home is the kitchen, and by observing how it is kept we can understand what the condition of the entire family must be. For example, if the refrigerator contains meat, eggs, milk and leftovers from several weeks ago, and if it has a stale odor when we open the door, we can surmise that the people eating in that house must be experiencing many sicknesses and difficulties.

The colors that people choose for the interiors of their homes also reveal much about their conditions. Each color has a unique quality and influence upon our lives. A red-colored room, for example, creates a more hot, unsettled, and irritable feeling, while blue creates the opposite, a feeling of calm and relaxation. This is because each color emits a different wavelength or vibration. Air circulation is also very important. A sick person should not rest in a room with poor circulation, as a stagnant environment is not conducive to health. To promote health and well-being, our home and surroundings should be as simple and natural as possible.

3. Ancestral and Spiritual Diagnosis

A. Ancestral Diagnosis. This type of diagnosis includes the ability to see and interpret various characteristics that are inherited from parents, grandparents, and ancestors. Fig. 9 illustrates the relationship that each of us has to our respective ancestors.

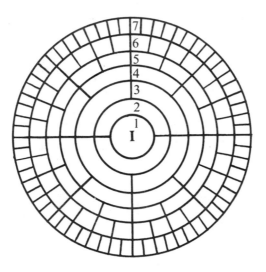

Fig. 9. *The relationship that we have to our ancestors is illustrated in the above mandala. This chart depicts seven generations, counting ourselves (I).*

We stand at the center of this chart (I) and originally exist in the form of a fertilized ovum. The union of our father's sperm with an egg from our mother, represented by (2), begins this process. In turn, each of our parents receives this same influence from their parents (3), and each of our grandparents receives this influence from their parents (4), who in turn receive their parents' influence (5), and so on through (6) and (7). Each of us has two parents, four grandparents, eight great-grandparents, 16 great-great grandparents; their parents number 32, and theirs, 64. Counting ourselves, this totals seven generations. Each of our ancestors influences us to some degree. Those closer to us in time have a greater influence, while those who are farther removed have less. Of course, we can trace our lineage back to infinity itself, but for practical use, the influence of the last seven generations, counting ourselves, can be seen within the body.

For example, the right side of the face is generally more yang than the left side. Since the egg moves downward and is relatively compact, it is more yang, meaning that it is governed primarily by centripetal force. Conversely, sperm are more active, move upward and are created through a process of differentiation, and are therefore more yin. The influence that we receive from our mother is more yang, and is reflected in the right side of the face, whereas our father's more yin influence can be seen in the left side. In the same way, the lines on the right palm reveal the influence received by the mother, while those on the left represent the father's influence.

Once this is understood, we are able to formulate a general picture of person's parents—what type of people they were, what were their favorite foods, and who was strongest. Everyone's face is unbalanced, one side always being more contracted than the other. This means that one side is smaller and the nose will often curve in that direction. When a person speaks, the side of the mouth which is on the more contracted side will be more active. The more yang, contracted side of the face also indicates which parent was more active.

We can also determine the condition of our parents by observing the palms of our hands. (See Fig. 10.) The three major lines in the palm reveal the condition of the three major bodily systems. The "life-line" corresponds to the digestive and respiratory systems; the "line of intellect" to the nervous system; and the "line of emotion" to the circulatory and excretory systems. If these systems are natively strong and healthy, all of these lines will be deep and clear. The digestive system line should be long and unbroken. If the lines on your right palm are stronger, your mother was a more active person. If your left palm is better, your father was stronger.

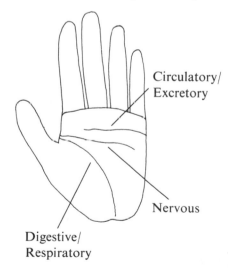

Circulatory/
Excretory

Nervous

Digestive/
Respiratory

Fig. 10. *The three major lines on the palm reveal the condition of the principal bodily systems. The lines on the right palm correspond to the influence received from the mother, while those on the left reveal the father's influence.*

We can further subdivide the face in order to determine the condition of a person's grandparents. (See Fig. 11.) When we divide each side in half, the inside half shows the more yang influence of the grandmother, while the outer half shows the grandfather's more yin influence. The right side would show the conditions of the maternal

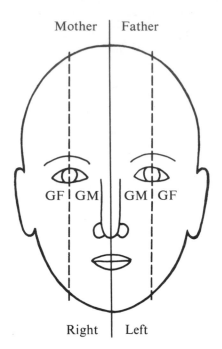

Mother | Father

GF | GM | GM | GF

Right | Left

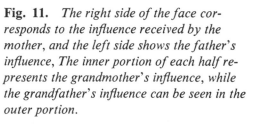

Fig. 11. *The right side of the face corresponds to the influence received by the mother, and the left side shows the father's influence, The inner portion of each half represents the grandmother's influence, while the grandfather's influence can be seen in the outer portion.*

grandparents, while on the left, we can see the paternal grandparents.

Careful observation of the eyes shows that each corner is different. In Fig. 12. we can see that one of the corners is open or expanded (1); another is very tight (2); one is more undefined (3); while another is moderately tight (4). The inner corner of the right eye shows the condition of the maternal grandmother, and since, in this case, it is the most yang or tight, she was the strongest grandparent. The outer corner of the right eye, which reflects the condition of the maternal grandfather, is the most loose or expanded, thus of the four grandparents his condition was the weakest. The left eye shows that the father's parents were in between.

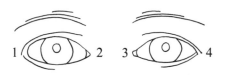

1   2   3   4

Fig. 12. *The corners of the eyes reveal the condition of someone's grandparents. In the illustration at left, the maternal grandmother was the strongest, or the most yang, of the grandparents.*

Each of us has 64 ancestors extending back seven generations. Dividing this number in half, we obtain the number 32. This correlates, in the upper region of the body, to our 32 teeth. In the lower part of the body, it correlates to the number of spinal vertebrae. Each of our teeth and vertebrae corresponds to one of our ancestors. To understand this more clearly, let us see how these parts of our body develop during the embryonic stage. (See Fig. 13.)

The inner spiral of the body (A) develops into the digestive and respiratory systems, while the outer spiral (B) eventually becomes the nervous system. Thirty-two teeth develop at the end of this digestive spiral, while a similar number of vertebrae develop along the spiral of the nervous system. During the period of embryonic development, the brain and nervous system occupy a peripheral, or yin, position,

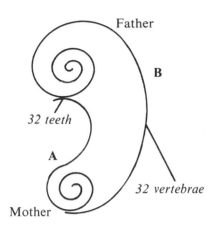

Father

B

32 teeth

A

Mother

32 vertebrae

Fig. 13. *The inner spiral of the body (A) later develops into the yin digestive system, while the peripheral spiral becomes the more yang nervous system (B).*

and because of this, carry the father's more yin influence. Of course, both parents influence our entire body, but in this instance the father's influence predominates. Conversely, the mother's more yang influence is centered predominantly in the digestive and respiratory systems, which occupy a more central, or inward position. If a man has a strong nervous system and good thinking power, his children will usually inherit this characteristic, unless, of course, they spoil themselves by eating improperly. In a related fashion, if a woman is natively strong and active, with a powerful digestive and respiratory system, her children should also enjoy this advantage.

Each of the 32 vertebrae reflects the influence of our 32 ancestors spanning seven generations on our father's side, while each tooth corresponds to the same ancestors on our mother's side. These influences also appear in other areas of the body. For example, the more yang, compacted organs reflect the influence of our mother's ancestors, and the more yin, hollow organs reflect the influence of our father's ancestors. These relationships correlate precisely with those studied in the science of genetics. In other words, the influence which is passed from generation to generation through the transfer of DNA correlates to that which is passed on through the mechanism of yin and yang.

B.   Rei-Sō: (靈相) Spiritual Diagnosis.   In Japanese, the word *Rei* means "spirit." This type of diagnosis involves being able to perceive the influences exerted by people who have died. To explain this in modern terms, we may interpret the term "spirit" to mean "vibration," "energy," or "consciousness." Let us consider several types of influence that human beings receive from the world of spirit so as to better understand this type of diagnosis. Many of us have an image of an ideal person. We may think, "I would like to be like Socrates, Jesus, Lao Tsu, Albert Schweitzer," or some other person. As a result, we often carry an image of that person which affects our consciousness and our life orientation. This is one type of spiritual influence. Another has to do with the attachment that we may have to people who were closely associated with us in life but who have died. If you had a special relationship with a particular person, such as a parent, ancestor, or close friend who has now passed away, his or her spirit will often become attached to you. A large number of people are influenced by spirits of this type, which you may also call "ghosts."

For example, several years ago a desperate young man came to see me. Not only was his physical condition poor, but he was suffering from emotional and psychological disorders as well. His condition was so poor that as soon as he entered, the atmosphere of the room became dark and depressing. Both of his parents had died, and his brothers and sisters were either suffering from mental illness or had already experienced an untimely death. When I inquired about his ancestors, he replied that they had been slave traders in colonial America. Since this young man's ancestors were involved in such an occupation, their negative influence was transferred from generation to generation and was the cause of his family's unhappiness. In order to purify his condition, this young man began to eat macrobiotically and to pray to his ancestors, extending his appreciation to them as well as his sincere apologies on their behalf to the wandering spirits of the people whom they forced into slavery. After one year, he became very happy, strong, and healthy.

Wandering spirits appear over the shoulders. If they are seen over the left shoulder, they are either male spirits, such as a deceased husband, or are among the father's ancestors. When they appear over the right shoulder, they are either female spirits or are among the mother's ancestors.

As the case of the young man illustrates, our health may depend on whether we can make our spiritual condition clean by pacifying these wandering spirits. Prayer, self-reflection, and self-resurrection—changing the quality of our blood, cells, and entire being—are necessary to achieve this. Our consolation of unhappy spirits should ultimately extend beyond those directly influencing us to the entire realm of unhappy or deluded entities. Many people have suffered throughout mankinds' long history, and our modern civilization has literally been built upon the sacrifice and suffering of an untold number of people. Unless we begin to change this through the above methods, our civilization will produce great unhappiness and will end tragically.

4. Sō-Sō: (想相) Diagnosis by Thought and Image

The word Sō can be translated as "image," "thought," or "consciousness." This method of diagnosis has to do with the ability to see and understand the type of thoughts or images that a person has. Past memory and future vision comprise the two main poles of consciousness. Future thinking, which is yin, arises more in the front brain, whereas memories, which are more yang, arise primarily in the back brain. (See Fig. 14.) Each type of thinking is activated by different types of food. For example, if we eat foods such as honey, sugar, spices, salad, and fruits, we activate the more yin front portion of the brain. This leads to the development of futuristic ideas. On the other hand, if we are consuming plenty of yang foods like steak, salt, eggs, and others, we begin to activate the back part of the brain. People with this type of condition are often concerned with maintaining traditions.

Thoughts occur in the form of vibrations or wave lengths, including alpha and beta waves. When we think about the future, vibrations appear toward the front of the head. When we think of the past, vibrations appear more toward the back of the head, and images of the present take the form of vibrations around the center of the head on either side. The frequency or intensity of these vibrations is determined by the type of image that we create. For example, when we practice meditation or what

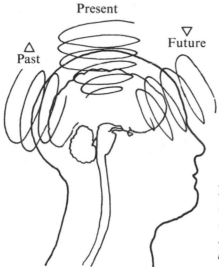

Fig. 14. *Future thinking is generated in the more yin cortex while memory arises in the brain's rear section which is more yang. Images of the present are created in the brain's central regions.*

is called "non-thinking," the vibrations around the head become very quiet. However, as our thoughts become active or vigorous, such as when we think about the opposite sex, our business, or financial position, or about some type of struggle or conflict, the vibrations around the head become correspondingly active and intense.

If your condition is sensitive, you can detect these vibrations by applying your hand to the different regions of the head, to sense which areas of the brain are active, and to what degree. It is even possible to detect these vibrations without touching; in other words, to actually see what type of thoughts a person is having. A person with this ability knows whether someone is lying or telling the truth, or whether what he or she is saying is different from what he or she is thinking.

To practice this method of diagnosis, it is necessary to use what is called "non-focussing" vision, which is similar to the type of vision that newborn infants have before developing the ability to focus upon specific objects. Our breathing should be very quiet, with the out-breath being four to five times longer than the in-breath. Begin to unfocus your eyes during the out-breath.

5. Diagnosis by Expression

All forms of expression reveal our condition, since our habits, speech, movements, writing, and other day-to-day modes of expression are the result of the foods we have been eating. For example, suppose someone shakes his foot while sitting in a cross-legged position. This is the opposite of a condition like polio, and is caused by the overconsumption of yang foods. Sleepwalking offers another example. This condition is also caused by the consumption of too many yang foods, and can be cured in one week by eliminating animal products and consuming foods of vegetable quality.

6. Diagnosis by Character and Nature

This type of diagnosis is similar to the above, and is based on the ability to understand what personal preferences, such as the type of clothing that people wear, the type of hobbies they have, the type of books they read, reveal about their condition. Another important aspect of this diagnosis is based on the understanding of basic character differences which result from different birth dates. This is also known as "astrological diagnosis."

One aspect of astrological diagnosis is based on the constitutional differences resulting from the season of birth. For example, someone born in May was conceived in August, and their embryonic development was spent predominantly during the colder months of winter, during which time their mother was probably eating a more yang diet—more cooked food, more salt, and possibly a higher percentage of animal food. As a result, this person's basic constitution is relatively yang. On the other hand, a person born in November, which is the opposite time of the year, began his embryonic life around February, passing through nine months of development during the spring, summer, and fall. Since their mother would naturally eat a more yin diet during this period, this person would have a more yin constitution.

In general, people born during the spring and summer, from March 21 to September 21, have more yang constitutions, while those born during the fall and winter, from September 21 to March 21, are natively more yin. Those born in June are the most yang, while persons born in December are the most yin. More yang persons tend to be more physically or socially active, while those who are more yin tend to involve themselves in intellectual or artistic pursuits.

7. Bo-Shin: (望診) Visual Diagnosis

This type of diagnosis is known in oriental medicine as *Bo-Shin*, and is based on the ability to understand the internal condition of the body by seeing its surface features. This art was widely practiced in ancient times, but, after several thousand years, has been largely forgotten. However, this ancient art is now being revived, and an increasing number of people have studied and are using it.

At the basis of visual diagnosis is the understanding of the various complementary and antagonistic relationships existing within the human body, such as that between (1) the upper and lower regions of the body, (2) the front and back of the body, (3) the left and right sides of the body, (4) the periphery of the body and the inside, and (5) the various parts of the body to the body as a whole.

A. The Upper and Lower Regions of the Body.   The upper region of the body refers to the area above the neck, while the lower region refers to that below the neck. For convenience, we will call the former the "head" and refer to the latter as the "body." In terms of structure, the head is compact and solid, and therefore yang, while the body is more large or expanded, and therefore yin. Since yin and yang are the inverse of each other, what exists in one exists in the other in an opposite form. In terms of the human body, what exists in the head in a more compacted form also exists in the body, but in an opposite, or expanded form. Therefore, the heart, lungs, intestines, and the other bodily organs have corresponding manifestations in the head, and we can see their condition by looking at the face.

The neck represents the center of the body, and from here, the head develops in an upward direction while the body develops downward. Therefore, the organs which

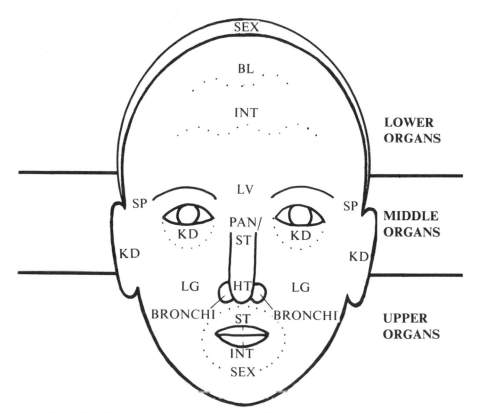

Fig. 15.   *The organs in the lower part of the body are reflected in the upper part of the face; those in the middle regions correlate to the middle of the face; while those in the upper region can be seen in the lower part of the face. The mouth reflects the condition of the digestive tract as well as the sexual organs.*

are located in the lower part of the torso appear in the upper region of the face, those in the central region appear in the central region of the face, and those in the upper region are reflected in the lower part of the face. (See Fig. 15.) Let us now examine these correlations in detail:

1. Lungs.   The lungs are reflected in the cheeks. Changes in their condition produce corresponding changes in the cheeks, particularly in regard to color. It is widely known that the cheeks take on a reddish color when the lungs become inflamed. Pimples on the cheeks indicate that fatty acid or mucus deposits are present in the lungs, while pale cheeks reveal a weak lung condition.

2. Heart.   The condition of the heart can be seen in the tip of the nose. A nose that is very enlarged indicates that the heart is likewise expanded, while a red nose shows that the heart is overworking, causing irregular blood pressure. A cleft in the center of the tip of the nose indicates a heart murmur. This condition is similar to a harelip, in which the right and left sides of the mouth did not fuse properly during the embryonic period. This is caused by the faulty diet of the mother, particularly a diet which is lacking in minerals. A cleft in the nose is less extreme than a harelip, and indicates that the left and right sides of the heart did not fuse properly, resulting in an irregular heartbeat.

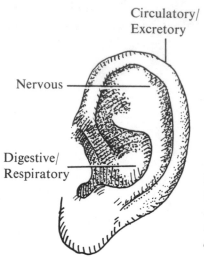

Fig. 16. *The inner ridge of the ear corresponds to the digestive and respiratory systems, the middle ridge to the nervous system, and the outer ridge to the circulatory and excretory systems.*

3. *Bronchi.*   The condition of the bronchi can be seen in the nostrils.

4. *Stomach and Pancreas.*   These organs, located more in the central part of the body, are reflected in the central and upper part of the nose.

5. *Kidneys.*   The kidneys, a pair of bean-shaped organs located in the central region of the back, correspond to the paired organs of the face—the eyes and ears. The ears also reflect the nature of a person's overall constitution. (See Fig. 16.) Until very recently, most people were born with large ears. Even today many persons over the age of 45 have large and well-developed ears which reflect a strong native constitution. However, many younger people have smaller ears, indicating that their kidneys are weak, as are their overall constitutions.

As we discussed in the section on ancestral diagnosis, the three major lines of the palm reveal the condition of the three major bodily systems. At the same time, these lines correlate to the three major ridges on the ear. The innermost ridge of the ear correlates with the lowest palm line, and shows the condition of the digestive and respiratory systems. The middle ridge corresponds to the middle palm line, and shows the condition of the nervous system. The outer ridge of the ear reflects the condition of the circulatory and excretory systems, and correlates to the upper palm line.

If the kidneys have become tight and contracted as a result of excessive salt intake, the region below the eyes often becomes dark. This symptom may also appear after excessive sexual activity. On the other hand, if this region becomes swollen or expanded—a condition commonly called "eyebags"—you can suspect that the kidneys are overworking as a result of the excessive intake of liquid. This is often accompanied by a condition in which the kidneys become swollen and waterlogged. Pimples in this region indicate that the kidneys have begun to accumulate fat and mucus, and if these deposits become hard, kidney stones are beginning to form.

6. *Liver and Spleen.*   The liver is more yang than the spleen, since it has a greater density, is reddish in color, and contains a larger number of red blood cells. As a result, it appears in the more contracted central region of the face, immediately above the nose. One or more vertical lines in this area indicate liver trouble. Since it is more yin, the spleen appears on both sides of the head in the region around the ends of the eyebrows. Discoloration in this region is an indication of spleen trouble.

7. *Intestines and Bladder.*   These organs, which are located in the lower portion of the body, appear in the upper region of the face, specifically in the forehead. If we drink excessively, we urinate more frequently, while at the same time we begin to perspire from the forehead. Lines or ridges in the forehead indicate trouble in these organs.

8. *Reproductive Organs.*   These organs are located in the lowest region of the body, and are therefore reflected in the hair, which is the uppermost part of the head. If someone's hair has many split ends, a yin condition, this indicates that his or her sexual ability is declining. At present, many people have fragile hair that breaks very easily. This also indicates that the reproductive and sexual functions are weak. Human hair should be strong and not easily breakable.

Each strand of hair contains a record of our past history. The tip of each hair reveals our past condition, while the root indicates our present condition. None of our hairs are uniform from the root to the tip. Some parts are thick, while others are more narrow; some regions may be lighter in color, while others are darker, and various regions of each hair are stronger or weaker. All of these variations reflect previous changes in our eating and in our physical condition. The fingernails also carry this history.

9. *The Digestive System.*   The mouth is the entrance of the digestive vessel. The condition of the entire digestive tract is reflected here, as is the condition of the anus and the sexual organs. (See Fig. 17.) Many people have swollen or protruding lower lips, which indicate that the lower part of the digestive vessel is also expanded. In other words, the intestines have become loose, producing an irregular bowel movement. An expanded upper lip indicates that the upper region of the digestive vessel, or the stomach, is not functioning properly.

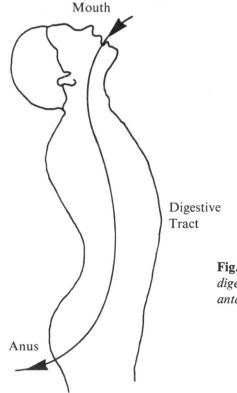

Mouth

Digestive
Tract

Fig. 17.   *The mouth is the beginning of the digestive system and is complementary-antagonistic to the anus.*

Anus

The inner portion of the lower lip shows the condition of the small intestine, while the outer section correlates to the large intestine. The duodenum corresponds to the corners of the mouth, or the area that is in between the upper and lower lips. Discolorations of the lips reveal corresponding problems in the digestive organs. For example, white patches on the lips indicate that mucus or fat deposits are accumulating in the intestines, while dark patches show the development of ulcers. In a similar way, the digestive condition can be seen in the tongue. The tip of the tongue corresponds to the lower region of the digestive tract, while the root of the tongue corresponds to the upper region.

The mouth and the area surrounding it also corresponds to the reproductive organs. It is in this region that men grow moustaches. A woman should not have a moustache. If she does, problems are developing in her sexual organs. Suppose that a woman has a moustache that is thicker on the right side. In this case, her right ovary would be the most affected.

B. The Front and Back of the Body.   The correlation between the front and back of the body represents another of the complementary and antagonistic relationships used in diagnosis. The principle of this relationship is simple—imbalances occurring in the front of the body, for example in the front internal organs, appear on the back as well. When we observe the condition of the spine or of the skin on the back, for example the manner in which the spine curves or the various types of markings or discolorations on the skin, we are able to determine which organs are disfunctioning.

C. The Right and Left Sides of the Body.   Besides helping us to understand the influences that we receive from our parents and ancestors, the body's left-right balance can also be used to understand the condition of the internal organs. (See Fig. 18.) For instance, let us assume that a person's right shoulder is higher, or more expanded. This indicates that the right lung is also more yin, or expanded, and is therefore weaker than the left lung. If the right lung is weaker, this influence is transferred to the opposite side of the diaphragm, meaning that the organs below the diaphragm on the left side are weaker. This condition is in turn transferred to the opposite leg, so that in this example, the right leg would tend to be weaker.

D. The Inside (Center) of the Body and the Periphery.   We cannot analyze the internal organs through direct observation without artificial measures, but it is possible to fully understand their condition by seeing their manifestations at the periphery of the body. When troubles occur inside the body, signs appear immediately at the periphery. These include symptoms like chipped fingernails, excessive body hair, skin markings like moles or beauty marks, and many others, all of which reveal past and present imbalances in the internal organs.

E. The Parts of the Body and the Body as a Whole.   We have already seen how this relationship works in the case of the ears and the palms of the hand. Let us now consider how the condition of the entire body can be understood by observing the whites of the eyes. By dividing the eye horizontally, we obtain an upper section, which corresponds to the organs in the upper region of the body, and a lower section, which corresponds to the organs in the lower region. When we divide the eye ver-

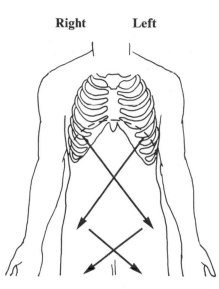

Right   **Left**

Fig. 18. *The right-left correspondences of the body cross at the diaphragm and again at the legs.*

tically, we obtain an inner and an outer half. The more yang inner section corresponds to the part of the body that is structurally more compact—the back or spinal region. Conversely, the outer, more yin section corresponds to the front of the body which is structurally more yin—soft and expanded. We can then divide the eye into twelve sections in order to determine more precisely the areas in which specific organs appear. These correlations appear in Fig. 19.

Bloodshot areas in specific parts of the eye indicate problems in the corresponding organs. For example, bloodshot in the region that corresponds to the brain means that the blood capillaries in this area are inflamed and expanded. Bloodshot in the area corresponding to the sexual organs indicates that the capillaries in these organs are expanded and may be overflowing with blood. In some cases, a woman will develop bloodshot in this area during menstruation, but this should disappear after the completion of her menstrual period. If this condition is constant, however, it is a symptom of chronic trouble in the sexual organs. Dark spots appearing in the upper region of the eye indicate the development of calcified stones in the sinuses; when seen in the lower region they signal the possible formation of kidney stones or ovarian cysts.

If the whites of the eyes become yellowish, the liver and gall bladder are malfunctioning. A dark color indicates kidney and bladder trouble, while a reddish color shows that the heart and small intestine are not working properly. As with the face, a gray color in the eyes indicates liver trouble, a pale color shows lung and large intestine trouble, and a green color shows the development of cancer. Cancer may also be reflected in the eyes as a transparency found in the area corresponding to the afflicted location in the body. Another common symptom is the appearance of white or yellow patches on the eyeball. If these appear on the lower part of the eyeball underneath the lower lid, it is an indication of fat and mucus in the lower part of the body, particularly around the sexual organs. In woman, this is an indication of a chronic vaginal discharge, while in men, it indicates prostate trouble.

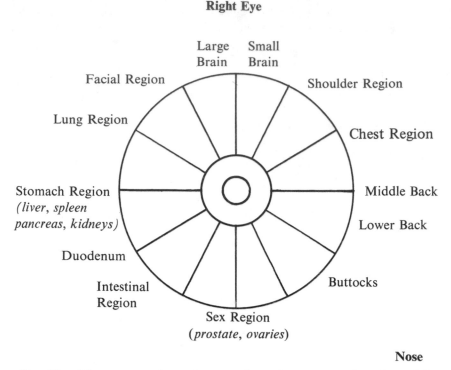

Fig. 19. *The correspondences between the major organs and sections of the body and the whites of the eyes.*

8. Bun-Shin: (聞診) Audio-Diagnosis

Bun-Shin is the ancient art of diagnosing a person's condition by the sound of his voice. If you listen to many voices, you will notice that some are very high-pitched; some are interrupted by frequent pauses; and some are watery, while others are unclear. All of these qualities reveal much about a person's condition. For example, a watery voice indicates kidney trouble, while speech that is interrupted by frequent pauses warns of heart problems. If someone's speech sounds heavy or stagnant, this is an indication that the lungs are coated with mucus. Any type of condition, such as kidney stones, fever, diarrhea, or constipation, will appear in the voice. Persons who are skilled in this art can understand someone's condition within 30 seconds after hearing his or her voice, even over the telephone.

We can also diagnose someone's condition by examining his handwriting. Everyone's handwriting is different, and by analyzing these differences, it is possible to determine the type of sickness a person has, which of his organs are strongest and which are weakest, and a variety of other conditions.

9. Diagnosis by Smell

Everyone has a unique body odor, according to the type of food eaten. In general, persons who eat well and who are healthy do not discharge much odor. The deodorant industry is a symptom of chaotic eating which creates strong odors as the body discharges toxins. Perfumes are more popular in western than in eastern countries, because people in the West tend to have a poorer condition which is reflected in stronger body odors.

An unpleasant body odor results from a diet that is high in meat and other animal products, as well as dairy food. Under normal circumstances, the carcass of an animal starts to putrefy immediately after it has been killed. Bacteria begin to multiply and an unpleasant odor soon develops. However, this is largely avoided through the modern techniques of freezing and chemical preservation. Meat, however, immediately starts to decay upon entering the digestive tract, and, upon reaching the intestines, the bacteria which are produced by this putrefaction begin to spread. This disrupts the normal functioning of the intestine, since these bacteria destroy the beneficial intestinal bacteria which synthesize B-Complex Vitamins and other necessary compounds.

The putrefaction of animal proteins in the intestines also produces an unpleasant odor, which is first apparent in the bowel movement. If these foods continue to be eaten, an unpleasant odor will spread to the underarms and other parts of the body.

This condition can be cured by eating primarily grains and vegetables, and by limiting the intake of animal products.

Various disorders in the internal organs produce specific types of odors. For example, a person with liver or gall bladder trouble will exude an oily or greasy smell. Someone with trouble in the heart and small intestine will give off a burnt smell, while spleen-pancreas or stomach troubles produce a roasting odor. Diseases of the lungs and large intestine, such as tuberculosis, coughing, and bronchitis, produce a smell that resembles fish, while trouble in the kidneys or bladder often results in a putrefying smell.

10. Meridian Diagnosis

The meridians are pathways of electromagnetic energy, and are not a part of any of the body's systems. Interestingly enough, western science and medicine were unaware of their existence until very recently, although they have been widely known and used in the Orient for the past five or six thousand years. Meridians occur universally in nature. For example, the lines on a leaf show the presence of meridians, as do the ridges of a cactus, and the earth itself contains a network of energy lines. The human body has 12 major pairs of meridians.

The meridians are created as a result of the electromagnetic charge existing between heaven and earth. (See Fig. 20.) The universe, or heaven, generates a centripetal force which enters the body through the hair spiral, while the expanding force produced by the earth's rotation enters through the genitals. After entering through the hair spiral, heaven's force charges the midbrain. This charge is distributed to the cells of the brain, and results in the formation of images and thoughts, similar to the way in which a television creates an image and sound. Proceeding downward, heaven's force charges the area deep inside the mouth, and results in the creation of the uvula. It also charges the root of the tongue, and passing downward, charges and vitalizes the vocal cords and thyroid and parathyroid glands.

Proceeding further, it charges the heart and surrounding area, resulting in the

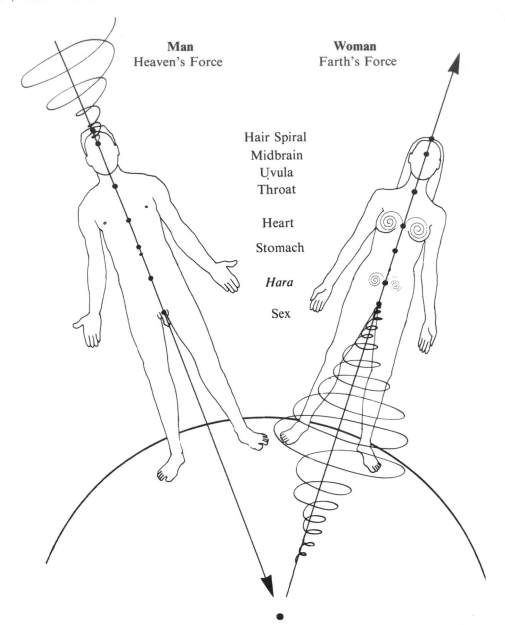

Man
Heaven's Force

Woman
Earth's Force

Hair Spiral
Midbrain
Uvula
Throat

Heart

Stomach

Hara

Sex

Fig. 20. *The major charging regions along the primary channel of heaven's and earth's forces, along with the sexual differentiation that is created by the predominance of either of these forces at particular locations. This main channel is the origin of the 12 pairs of meridians.*

continual expansion and contraction of this organ, as well as in the movements of breathing. The stomach is the next major region to be activated by heaven's force, and from there, energy is distributed to the liver, spleen, gall bladder, pancreas, and kidneys, stimulating their respective functions.

Heaven's force then charges the region deep inside the small intestine, known in the Orient as *hara*. This creates the rhythmic movements of both the small and large intestine, as well as the absorption of digested foodstuffs by the villi and the secretion of intestinal juice. Heaven's force exits from the body in the region of the sexual organs. In men, it creates here a second uvula-like organ known as the penis.

Of course, women also receive heaven's force, but this energy is superseded in the lower region of the body by earth's expanding force. As a result, women do not have a large "uvula" in the lower part of the body as men do, but instead have a smaller one known as the clitoris. At the same time, earth's upward-moving force creates the vagina and uterus, which are formed in an inward, upward direction in comparison to the male sexual organs. Earth's force continues upward to the *hara* region, where it collides with heaven's descending force, creating spirals known as the ovaries. Both forces collide again at the region of the heart, and the spirals created here form the breasts. Since earth's force is stronger in women, their voices tend to have a higher pitch. Also, women tend to develop longer hair, which grows in an upward direction on the head, while men usually have less head hair and more downward-growing body hair.

To summarize, women are charged more by earth's centrifugal, yin, expanding force; while men are influenced more by heaven's centripetal, yang, contracting force. This fundamental difference formed the basis of the traditional association of women with the earth and men with heaven. Naturally, different mental, physical and emotional tendencies arise out of these basic constitutional differences. Viewed from this perspective, we see that sex is simply the attraction of these two complemental forces to merge and create harmony.

The meridians are the supplemental channels which radiate outward from the main heaven-earth channel. A similar phenomenon occurs in apples, apricots, and other fruits, as well as in vegetables like squash and pumpkins. The ridges on the surface of a pumpkin outline the path of its meridians, or surface channels of electromagnetic current, while the outline of the main heaven-earth channel can be seen in the core.

In the human body, meridians channel electromagnetic current to and from each of the body's organs. While in the womb, our development takes the form of a spiral. The peripheral region of this spiral later becomes the spine and nervous system, while the inside or central region later becomes the front of the body. This highly-charged embryonic spiral receives a constant supply of energy from the environment, primarily in the form of 12 major currents which enter through the back. Upon reaching the most deep inner region of the body, this energy begins to condense and form smaller spirals of its own. These smaller spirals later develop into the various bodily organs, and from here, this energy is discharged through the front of the body. This discharge manifests primarily as a pair of upper and lower spirals which later develop into the arms and legs. These paths of discharge later become the meridians. (See Fig. 21.)

The first type of meridian diagnosis consists of examining each meridian for the purpose of correlating various skin discolorations with the condition of the corresponding organ. For example, many people have so-called "beauty marks" along the meridians. These show that at one time the person had some type of sickness in the corresponding organ which was accompanied by high fever. The beauty mark is a remnant of this, caused by the discharge of carbon produced by the burning of the fever.

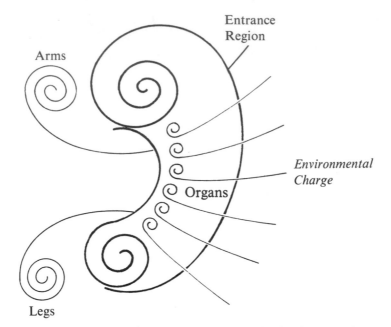

Arms

Entrance
Region

Environmental
Charge

Organs

Legs

Fig. 21. *Energy from the environment enters the developing embryo through the back, creates the internal organs, and exits through the front of the body along the arms and legs.*

Each finger and toe is connected to a meridian, and by examining them we are able to determine the condition of the corresponding organs. (See Fig. 22.) For example, curved fingers show an imbalance in the corresponding organ. If they curve away from the thumb, the imbalance is a result of excessive yin, while a curvature toward the thumbs is caused by excessive yang. Toes which are curled or twisted indicate potential weakness in their corresponding organs. If the second toe is longer than the first, the stomach is natively yin, and has a tendency to be weak.

The meridians can also be used to diagnose specific conditions such as cancer. The area around the base of the thumb on the inside of the hand corresponds to the digestive and respiratory systems. A green or blue color in this region is a sign of intestinal trouble, and possibly cancer. This area should be the same color as the rest of the palm.

In the case of colon cancer, the fleshy part of the outside of the hand between the thumb and index finger often takes on a green or bluish shade. This discoloration may also occur around other areas which lie on the large intestine meridian. In the case of small intestine cancer, a green or bluish color will often appear along the corresponding meridian, particularly around the outside of the hand between the wrist and the little finger. (See Fig. 23.)

Cancer in the liver or spleen will often appear as a greenish or bluish shade anywhere along their respective meridians. (The liver meridian runs from inside the first toe up along the inside of the leg, while the spleen meridian begins on the outside of the first toe and also continues along the inside of the leg.) With liver cancer, this discoloration often appears around the area below the knee, while persons with spleen or pancreatic cancer often develop it around the inside of the foot. If a person

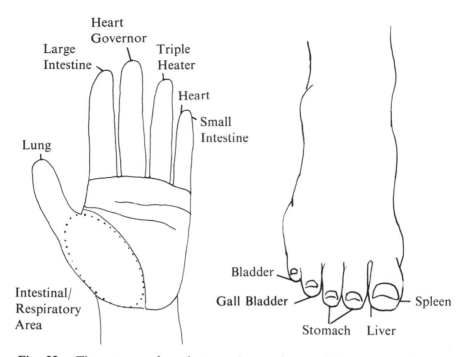

Fig. 22. *The correspondence between the meridians and the fingers and toes.*

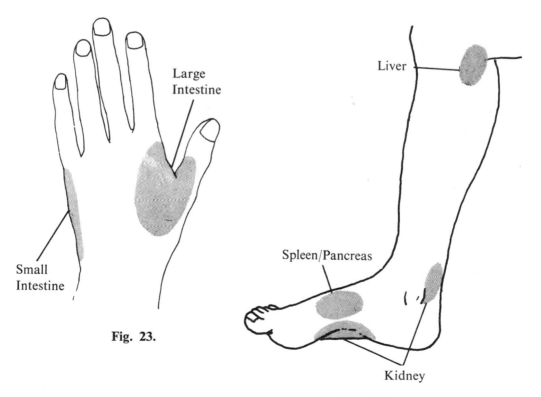

Fig. 23.

Fig. 24.

develops kidney cancer, a similar discoloration may occur anywhere along the corresponding meridian, which begins at the bottom of the foot and runs up along the inside of the leg. This often occurs around the arch of the foot or around the outside of the ankle. (See Fig. 24.)

The stomach meridian runs down the outside of the leg. It splits into two branches at a point located several inches below the knee. The main branch continues along the outside front of the leg to the second toe, while the secondary branch follows a similar path to the third toe. When stomach cancer develops, this area below the knee often becomes discolored. If the gall bladder becomes cancerous, this discoloration may occur on the outside of the foot, around the outside of the knee, or anywhere along this meridian, which runs down the outside of the leg to the fourth toe. Cancer of the bladder, uterus, prostate or sexual organs may produce discoloration along the bladder meridian. This meridian runs down the back of the leg to the fifth toe, and discoloration often appears on either side of the foot around the ankle. (See Fig. 25.)

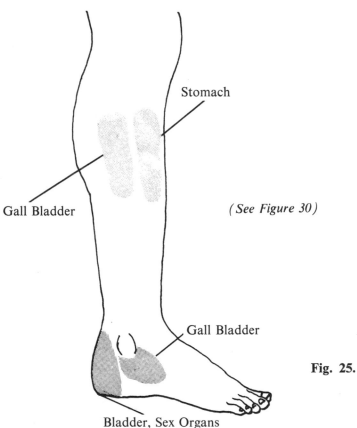

Stomach

Gall Bladder

(See Figure 30)

Gall Bladder

Fig. 25.

Bladder, Sex Organs

Another method of meridian diagnosis is based on the ability to detect subtle variations in the quality of the energy which passes along these channels. For example, when you hold your hand slightly above the skin and pass it along a meridian, you may feel very intense or strong vibrations over some regions, while over others, almost none at all. Acupuncture, massage, and other techniques of oriental medicine were used in cases like this to restore balance by activating the regions where energy was lacking, or drawing it out from the overactive areas.

Another type of meridian diagnosis involves using the fingers to probe directly along the meridian. Suppose that while diagnosing the lung meridian in this manner, you come to a region that is tight and painful. This indicates that mucus and fat deposits are starting to form in the lung, and that its overall condition is weakening. This technique can be applied to any of the meridians.

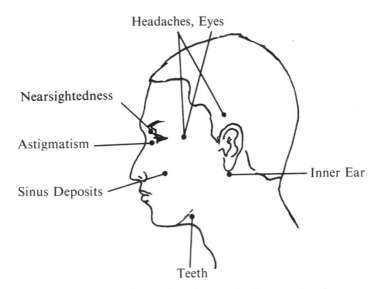

Fig. 26. *Major diagnosis points on the face and head.*

11. Shoku-Shin: (触診) Pressure-Point Diagnosis

Let us now study the major points along the meridians which can be used to diagnose the internal condition.

The point above the eyes, shown in Fig. 26, can be used to diagnose nearsightedness. If you feel pain when you press this point, you may have this condition. The point located on either side in the indented region above the nose can be used to diagnose astigmatism, or double vision. Pain here indicates the possibility of this condition. If you feel pain when the point located in the indented area of the center of each cheekbone is pushed, mucus is accumulating in your sinuses. The point in the indented region just below the earlobes can be used to determine the condition of the inner ear. If pain is felt here, deposits of mucus and fat are beginning to form, and hearing is starting to deteriorate.

Pain in the temple means that the brain is expanded, and that headaches may develop frequently. In many instances, people with headaches intuitively massage this area to obtain relief. This point can also be used to diagnose and treat eye problems. The point in the indented region of the jaw can be used to diagnose problems with the teeth. Pressure can also be applied to these points to help relieve the pain of a toothache.

On the front of the body, as shown in Fig. 27, the point located in the center of the breast bone, about 1½ inches above the area where the sternum and ribcage meet, is called *Dan-Chu*. This point can be used to diagnose the condition of the heart. If you feel pain when you press here, your heart is enlarged. If you feel pain when you push the points which are under the collarbone, you are suffering from lung trouble, while pain in the point located 1 to 1½ inches above the breastbone means that trouble is developing in the bronchi. This point is usually very sensitive in cases of bronchitis or asthma. To find the liver diagnosis points, follow the slanting inner side of the ribcage until you come to the indented areas illustrated in Fig. 27. If you feel pain when these points are pressed upward and inward, your liver has become expanded and hard, and is not functioning properly.

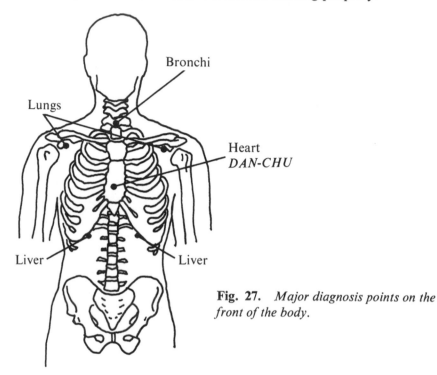

Fig. 27. *Major diagnosis points on the front of the body.*

If there is pain while pressing the points in the center of the palms, shown in Fig. 28, your circulation has become weak, possibly as a result of an excessive fluid intake. These points can also be used to diagnose the functioning of the sexual organs. The point located on the inside of either forearm around the elbow is on the lung meridian. Pain here indicates lung trouble. The large intestine diagnosis point lies on the outside of the hand in the fleshy part between the thumb and index finger. This point is known in the Orient as *Go-Koku.* The large intestine meridian continues up the arm, and contains another diagnosis point at the elbow. Pain in either of these points indicates problems in the large intestine.

The kidney diagnosis point is located on the bottoms of both feet as shown in Fig. 29. This point is called *Yu-Sen,* which means "bubbling spring," and is the beginning of the kidney meridian. Pain in this area indicates kidney trouble. On the insides of the legs, about 2½ inches above the anklebone, is a point called *San-In-Ko,* or "three-yin-junction." The meridians of the spleen and pancreas, liver, and kidney all meet at this point, which was traditionally used to diagnose and treat troubles in these organs, as well as in the sexual organs. (These organs are all yang —solid and compact—but their meridians are yin, hence the name *San-In-Ko.*) If

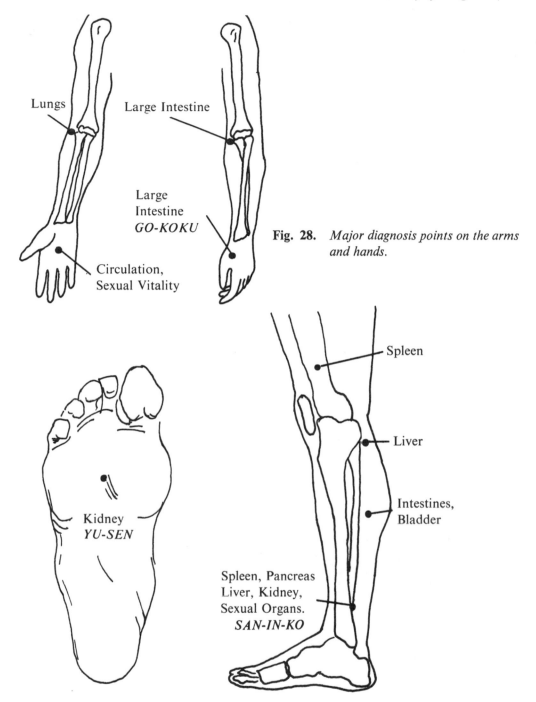

Lungs

Large Intestine

Large Intestine
GO-KOKU

Circulation,
Sexual Vitality

Fig. 28. *Major diagnosis points on the arms and hands.*

Kidney
YU-SEN

Spleen

Liver

Intestines,
Bladder

Spleen, Pancreas
Liver, Kidney,
Sexual Organs.
SAN-IN-KO

Fig. 29. *Major diagnosis points on the inside of the leg and foot.*

you feel pain when this point is pushed, among other problems, your sexual organs are becoming weak. Another important point is located further up the insides of the legs at the same level as the most expanded part of the calf. If this point is painful when pushed, it is an indication of trouble in the intestines and bladder, which often results from expansion or looseness caused by excessive eating and drinking.

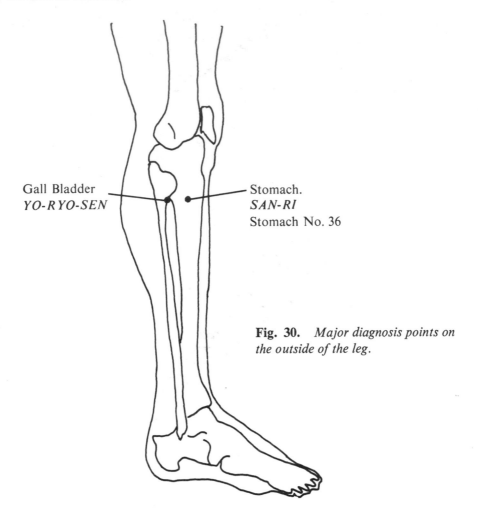

Gall Bladder
YO-RYO-SEN

Stomach.
SAN-RI
Stomach No. 36

Fig. 30. *Major diagnosis points on the outside of the leg.*

The liver diagnosis point is located on the inside of the leg below the knee, while the spleen-pancreas diagnosis point is located several inches above the knee against the inner part of the thighbone. Pain in either of these points indicates trouble in these organs.

There is a very well-known point located about three inches down from the bottom of the kneecap, in the area indicated in Fig. 30. Known as *San-Ri* (Stomach No. 36), this point is used to diagnose and treat stomach and overall digestive disorders. If there is tightness when this point is pushed, electromagnetic current is not flowing smoothly through the stomach meridian, which runs along the outside of the leg to the second and third toes. This can result in breathing and digestive difficulties, an inability to relax, and a tendency to tire easily.

Traditional oriental doctors relieved blockages in this point with needles, moxa (heat), or finger-pressure. If moxa is not available, then a cigarette can be used for the purpose of generating heat. To apply this method, called "cigarette moxa," bring a lit cigarette to about 1/3 of an inch above the point, while rotating it in a circular motion. When this becomes too hot, remove the cigarette, approach the point, and again remove when it becomes hot. This can be repeated three to five times. The gall bladder diagnosis point is located at the same level as *San-Ri* but about 1¼ inch more toward the outside of each leg. If pain is felt here, this organ is in trouble. Cigarette moxa can also be applied to this point, as well as to any of the points that we have studied, in order to release tightness or stagnation.

12. Pulse Diagnosis

In modern medicine, the pulse is used primarily to determine the condition of the heart and circulatory system. However, in oriental medicine, the pulses are used to gain a much more detailed picture of an individual's health. This refined type of pulse diagnosis can be used to judge the condition of each of the major organs. So as to better understand how this is possible, let us consider the relationship of the pulses to the universal cycle known in the Orient as the "Five Transformations," or *Go-Gyo*. This process was used to describe the order of change which governs all phenomena, and is one of the most fundamental concepts underlying the medicine, culture, and philosophy of the Orient.

Let us consider the progress of change within the world of matter. When gross or solid matter begins to expand, it changes into liquid, gas, and then plasma, which is familiar to us in the form of fire. From here, an opposite process occurs, as matter begins to solidify and condense back into the solid stage. This process is endless, and involves the transformation of matter into energy, and energy into matter. A familiar example is the cycle in which water evaporates, condenses, falls as precipitation, pools on the surface of the earth, and again evaporates. Ancient people assigned familiar names to each of these stages in order to facilitate an understanding of this universal process. The plasmic state was referred to as *fire*; the state of solidification, *soil*; the stage of gross matter, *metal*; the liquid stage, *water*; and the gaseous state was called *wood*. These stages were understood as being manifestations of the eternal cycle between expansion and contraction, or yin and yang, which occurs throughout the universe. (See Fig. 31.)

Ancient people were also aware of the subtle differences in the type of energy nourishing and sustaining each of the body's organs. In some cases, this energy is thick and condensed, while in others it is more diffused or expanded. This energy was classified as follows in terms of the five transformations:

1. Wood: This type of energy is expanding or outward-moving, and corresponds to the liver and gall bladder.

2. Fire: This type of energy has a dual nature. For example, matter, in the process of decomposing into energy, passes through the stage of plasma. This was known in oriental medicine as the stage of *primary fire*, and corresponds in the body to the heart and small intestine. At the same time, when energy begins to condense into matter, it too passes through the plasmic stage. Known as *secondary fire*, two of the body's comprehensive functions—the Heart Governor and Triple Heater— were classified in this category. The Heart Governor is the name given to the bodily functions which regulate the internal flow of blood and body fluid, while the Triple Heater refers to the functions which convert digested foodstuff into caloric energy.

3. Soil: This represents the stage in which energy is beginning to condense and solidify. This type of energy nourishes the spleen, pancreas, and stomach.

4. Metal: This type of energy is more thick and condensed, and corresponds to the lungs and large intestine.

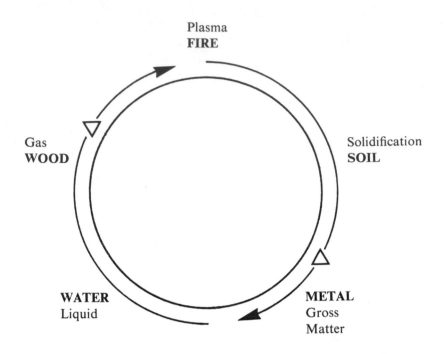

Fig. 31. *The Five Transformations—Go-Gyo* (五行).

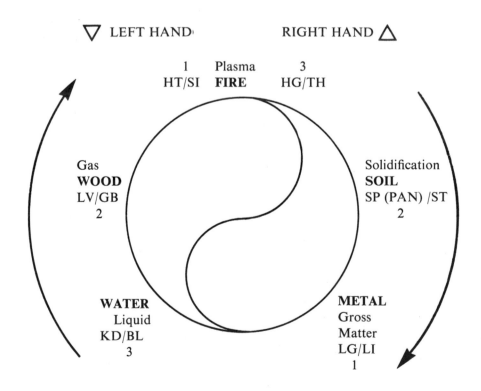

Fig. 32. *The Five Transformations and their corresponding organs and pulses.*

5. *Water:* This type of energy corresponds to the bladder and kidneys.

The stages of plasma, gas, and liquid represent the more yin tendencies within this cycle. (See Fig. 32.) The heart and small intestine, which correspond to primary plasma (1), represent the most yin of these tendencies. The liver and gall bladder, which correspond to wood, or gaseous matter (2), represent a medium-yin tendency, while the stage of water, or liquid matter (3), which corresponds to the kidneys and bladder, is the least yin of the three. The opposite, or more yang tendencies in this cycle are represented by the stages of metal, soil, and secondary plasma. The most condensed of these is metal (1), which corresponds to the lungs and large intestine. The spleen, pancreas and stomach, which correspond to the stage of soil (2), have a medium-yang nature, while the least yang of these is the stage of secondary plasma (3), which corresponds to the Heart Governor and Triple Heater.

The pulses of the organs which correspond to the more yin transformations appear on the primarily yin, left wrist, while on the more yang, right wrist, we can detect the organs which correspond to the yang transformations. In both cases, the pulses appear in the order of greatest yang to least yang, and greatest yin to least yin, in accordance with their correspondence to the five transformations. (See Fig. 33.)

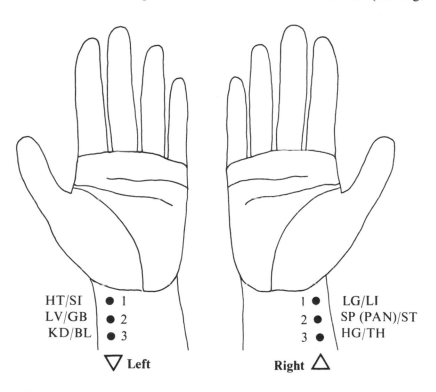

Fig. 33. *Pulse correspondences on the left and right hands. The pulses illustrated are those for men; in the case of women, the yin transformations appear on the right wrist, while the yang transformations appear on the left.*

Among the organs appearing on the left hand, the heart, liver, and kidneys are more solid and compact; while the small intestine, gall bladder, and bladder are more hollow and expanded. On the right hand, the lungs, spleen, and Heart Governor are more condensed; while the large intestine, stomach, and Triple Heater functions are expanded. However, the more yang, compacted organs are nourished by slower-moving, less active energy which is yin, while the yin, hollow organs are nourished by a yang, fast-moving and active type of energy. Therefore, the more active, surface pulses reflect the condition of the yin, or hollow organs, while the deeper, more subtle pulses reflect the yang, compacted organs. (See Fig. 34.)

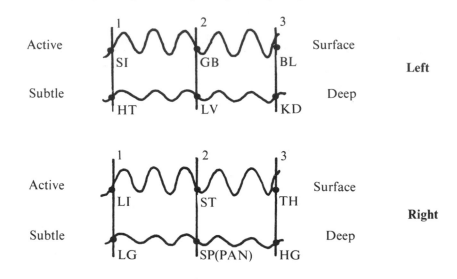

Fig. 34. *Positions of the surface and deep pulses.*

When taking the pulse, place your index, middle, and ring fingers next to each other on the three points indicated in Fig. 33. With your fingers in position, apply light pressure to each point in order to detect the superficial, or surface pulse. To find the deep pulse, press each point deeply, almost to the extent that you cannot press further. After checking both the superficial and deep pulses on one wrist, repeat the same procedure on the opposite wrist. There are subtle variations in the pulses which enable us to diagnose a variety of conditions in the organs. Some pulses may feel "jumpy," while others may seem hard or rigid. Some may be irregular, while others will be even and steady. Traditional practitioners of pulse diagnosis were able to identify about 140 different symptoms with this method.

The flow of energy is more active in the superficial pulses, and thus, they are usually detectable even in cases of serious sickness. In many instances, however, the deep pulses cannot be felt, even when a person appears to be healthy. Among practitioners of oriental medicine, it was commonly understood that if four out of the six deep pulses could not be felt, a patient had no hope of recovery, except through dietary adjustment. A more common condition is for several of the deep pulses to be undetectable, or for the pulses to beat in an irregular manner. Such indicators reveal precisely which organs are not functioning properly.

The pulses can also be used to understand the overall body condition. In general, the surface pulses reveal the general condition of *ki* flow which energizes the organs, while the deep pulses reveal the condition of the organs themselves. In between these is a third pulse which reveals the condition of the blood which nourishes each pair of organs. To detect this pulse, touch each point lightly, and then deeply, and then apply a medium pressure. By pressing the first point on the left hand in this manner, we can detect the condition of the nourishment passing via the bloodstream to both the heart and small intestine.

13. Diagnosis by Questioning

In this type of diagnosis we determine a person's condition by asking such questions as where he feels pain, if he has any abnormal symptoms, where he was born, when he was born, what type of family background he comes from, what type of foods he is eating, and others. The answers help us form a complete picture of an individual's state of health.

14. Diagnosis According to Discharge

This type of diagnosis includes body odor and voice diagnosis. Along with these, the color, odor, and texture of the bowel movement and urine can be used to form a diagnosis. A healthy bowel movement is solid, long, and dark gold in color. In the Orient, this color is described as "old gold." Urine should be somewhat lighter in color, or as it is referred to in the Orient, "new gold." Both of these vary with our changing condition. For example, if we eat unbalanced food, often we will have diarrhea the following day. Too much salt will turn the urine into a darker color, while too little results in a much lighter color. If too much fluid is consumed, urination will become very frequent. Normally, we should urinate three to four times a day. More than this indicates that too much fluid is being consumed, while less means that not enough is being consumed.

15. Diagnosis by Touching General Areas of the Body

By touching the shoulders, neck, forehead, hair, hands, feet, and other parts of the body, we can tell whether a person is tight or loose, dry or watery, warm or cold, oily or normal, as well as many other external appearances which reflect our internal condition.

16. Abdominal Diagnosis

It is possible to determine the condition of all of the major organs by applying pressure to their corresponding regions on the abdomen. (See Fig. 35.) The area located in the center of the abdomen, above the navel, corresponds to the heart and small intestine. The condition of the lungs and large intestine can be judged at the point to the right of the navel, while the left side reflects the condition of the liver and gall bladder. The area below the navel shows the condition of the kidneys and bladder, while the condition of the spleen, pancreas, and stomach appears in the central region around the navel.

To practice this method, have the person that you wish to examine lie comfortably on his or her back with raised knees. Ask him to breathe deeply, and, on the out-breath, press deeply but gently into the area that you are examining. If the organs are in a healthy condition, a normal pulse is felt when the corresponding regions

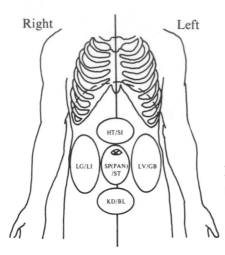

Right   Left

HT/SI

LG/LI   SP(PAN)/ST   LV/GB

KD/BL

Fig. 35. *The regions of the abdomen which can be used to diagnose specific organs.*

are pressed. If the organs are in poor condition, a larger, throbbing pulse will be felt, as well as hardness or tightness. The person will also experience pain when pressure is applied.

Appendix

Practical Diagnosis

Let us summarize our study of diagnosis with the following practical illustrations of how it can be used:

1. If a single symptom appears in a particular location, always check the place that is opposite to it. For example, if someone has pain in the shoulder, check the complementary and antagonistic region, which in this case would be the intestines. In many cases, shoulder pain is the result of an intestinal disorder. The relationship between the sinuses and the sexual organs offers another example. In many cases, mucus deposits in the sinuses indicate a similar problem in the sex organs, which may result in prostate trouble or vaginal discharges.

2. If the symptoms are multiple, for example, a headache plus ear difficulty, or nausea plus diarrhea, and pain in some area, check the meridians so as to understand the way in which the symptoms are interconnected. A problem such as this may involve only one or perhaps several meridians.

3. When head or facial troubles develop, always check the intestinal condition, as well as the related intestinal points on the hand. Conversely, if primary symptoms appear in the intestines, this will usually produce some type of head or facial disorder. For example, if the intestines are clogged because of constipation, excess will often rise and cause pimples, eye troubles, headaches, and other similar problems. Disorders such as these may also be the result of menstrual difficulties.

4. In cases of skin disease, check the internal condition through pressure-point, eye, or another form of diagnosis. The body's peripheral or surface condition always reflects the condition of the organs and other internal features.

5. If a person suffers from depression, check the mental and emotional as well

as physical condition, by using any of the methods included in spiritual and image and thought diagnosis. If someone is irritable, uneasy, and changes his mind often, check the balance between his father and mother. This tendency is often the result of an imbalance between parents.

6.   Someone who is very talkative can be diagnosed through audio diagnosis, while visual diagnosis can be used for someone who tends to be quiet. If someone is very active, base your diagnosis on his motion, expression, and mannerisms. If a person is unexpressive and not responsive to your questioning, you can diagnose the quality of his thoughts and images, while pressure-point, pulse, or abdominal diagnosis are effective in cases where someone is confined to bed.

Giving Advice

After we understand the nature of someone's problem through any of the above methods, the next step is to offer guidance as to how the problem can be overcome. The basic types of guidance or advice can be summarized as follows:

1.   Advice for the relief of symptoms.   This may require the recommendation of ginger compresses, taro plasters, and other external applications, as well as massage, moxibustion, palm healing, and other types of treatment. These treatments should be simple, natural, inexpensive, and should not produce side effects. Therefore, as much as possible, we should avoid the use of artificial medications.

2.   Advice for the relief of sickness by eliminating the cause.   As an example, let us consider a case in which a person with cancer suffers pain and water retention in the abdomen. A taro potato plaster would be helpful to relieve the pain, while a buckwheat plaster would be effective in reducing the abdominal swelling. However, since cancer results from an unhealthy blood and general bodily condition, these treatments will not actually eliminate the disease. For this, the person must restore the quality of the blood and cells through proper eating. In many cases, specific treatments or external applications are unnecessary, and should be used only when someone is experiencing pain or discomfort. However, proper diet should always form the basis of any type of program for the relief of sickness.

3.   Advice for permanent release from all difficulties and troubles.   The aim of this type of advice is to guide a person toward changing his way of life and thinking. A person who offers advice of this kind is no longer only a doctor or a healer, but also serves as a teacher of the proper way of life, which includes the practice of *self-reflection.*

For more detailed information on the above, as well as other, methods of diagnosis, please refer to the *How to See Your Health: The Book of Oriental Diagnosis* and *The Book of Dō-In: Exercise for Physical and Spiritual Development* by Michio Kushi, published by Japan Publications, Inc.

CHAPTER FOUR

The Digestive System

The digestive system occupies a more central position in the developing embryo, and therefore attracts more yin fats and proteins among the nutrients supplied by the mother's blood. As a result, the digestive system has a more hollow and expanded structure at birth. The digestive system is created in the form of an expanding spiral, which radiates outward from the central region known as the *hara*. Located about three fingers below the navel, deep within the small intestine, this region is one of the vital centers of the body, and is possibly one of the principal sites of red blood cell formation. This region is known in the Orient as *Ki-Kai*, or "sea of *ki*."

The digestive system should preferably be long, and should always be kept warm. It was for this reason that Orientals developed the *hara maki*, a special cotton wrapper worn around the abdomen.

The digestive system is counterbalanced by the nervous system. (See Fig. 36.) This system originally occupies a more peripheral position and during pregnancy attractes the yang nutritional components such as minerals and more yang proteins from the mother's blood. As a result, its structure at birth is compacted, shorter, and harder. The digestive system attracts and processes a more yang type of food in the form of physicalized, or material food. On the other hand, the nervous system processes a more yin type of food in the form of waves or vibrations. In between these two is the circulatory system, which includes the lymphatic and excretory systems. In terms of yin and yang, we can say that this third system is balanced. The respiratory system can be considered as a part of the digestive system. In terms of structure, it is compact and solid, and it attracts yin oxygen and discharges the more yang carbon dioxide. The digestive and respiratory systems complement each other in both structure and function. The former is structurally yin and processes yang food, while the latter is yang and handles yin in the form of gases.

The Physiology of Digestion

Food enters the body through the mouth and moves both spirallically and up-and-down in the process of chewing. (See Fig. 37.) Saliva normally has a pH factor of 7.2, which means that it is slightly alkaline before descending through the esophagus. In the stomach, gastric juices are secreted by 30 to 40 million gastric glands. There are two major gastric juices: (1) *pepsin*, which is secreted by round-shaped, yang gastric glands; and (2) *hydrochloric acid*, which is secreted by more yin, triangular-shaped cells located in the upper portion of the stomach. In general, gastric juice has a pH range of 0.9 to 1.5, meaning that it is a very strong acid. The influence of the digestive secretions alternate between alkaline and acid according to the following pattern:

—Mouth: alkaline
—Stomach: acid

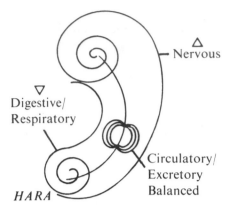

Fig. 36. *The spirallic formation of the human embryo, including the formation of the major bodily systems.*

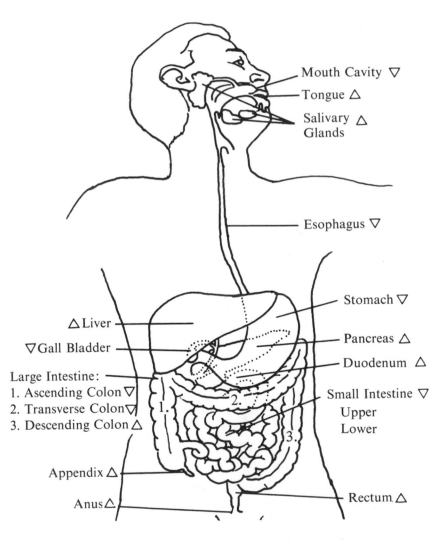

Fig. 37. *The Digestive System according to yin and yang.*

—Pancreas and Duodenum: alkaline

—Small Intestine: acid

Broken-down food particles are absorbed by the villi, found in the small intestine and duodenum. Villi are most numerous in the upper region of the small intestine (jejunum). Duodenal villi have a broader shape and a greater capacity to absorb alkaline substances. The villi in the small intestine are smaller and better suited to absorb acidic substances.

If we consume a strong yin like aspirin, alcohol, or refined sugar, absorbtion immediately begins in the mouth, due to the salty or alkaline nature of saliva. Refined bread or flour products are absorbed in the stomach, whereas whole grains, especially when cooked with salt, are not absorbed until they reach the villi. When a particular food is absorbed by the villi, its transformation into blood cells occurs smoothly. However, foods absorbed before reaching the villi, enter the body fluid prematurely, and produce a thinner quality of blood and lymph liquid. Therefore, to maintain health, our diet should be based primarily on foods which undergo the normal process of absorption by the intestinal villi.

When alkaline quality food enters the stomach, balance is achieved through the secretion of yin acids. This acidized food then travels to the duodenum where it is exposed to alkaline juices before moving to the small intestine, which secretes acid. The most important factor in proper digestion is whether or not food has been properly alkalized before it reaches the stomach. This is accomplished primarily through proper chewing, without which the digestive juices in the stomach, duodenum, and small intestine will not be secreted.

Carbohydrates are broken down in the mouth, by the action of saliva. In the stomach, the digestion of carbohydrates continues, but the acids secreted here function basically in the digestion of proteins. Fats are digested primarily in the duodenum, while in the intestines, a final breakdown of all foodstuffs takes place. This process is completed by the action of various intestinal micro-organisms which can be classified into two general groups:

1. The yin group of bacteria serves to decompose all foodstuffs into their most basic compounds. They act, for example, to break proteins down into amino acids.
2. The yang bacterial group serves to synthesize chemical compounds such as enzymes and vitamins.

Vegetable-quality foods do not easily putrefy and therefore do not usually disrupt the beneficial functioning of the intestinal bacteria. However, animal proteins start to decomposed as soon as the animal has been killed. This process in somewhat offset by refrigeration or by the addition of preservatives, but it resumes as soon as the animal protein is eaten, and is usually well underway by the time these foods reach the intestines. Putrefaction can be offset if animal proteins are eaten only occasionally and in small quantities, or if they are eaten along with plenty of vegetables. However, when they are eaten regularly, or in large quantities, the bacteria produced by this putrefaction remain in the intestines and disrupt the functioning of its beneficial micro-organisms.

In oriental medicine, the heart and small intestine and the lungs and large intestine were treated as pairs of organs. It was recognized that a problem in one organ always indicated some malfunction in the other. The proper functioning of the intestines is of vital importance to the overall health of the body, and if they are not working well, the activity of the heart, lungs, and other major organs will not proceed smoothly. The intestines are also closely related to the brain. The ridges in the brain are proportional in number and depth to those in the intestines, and both are composed of a similar type of tissue. Like the intestines, the condition of the brain should be more yang or compacted. When the brain cells begin to expand, schizophrenia or chaotic thinking result. Likewise, if the intestines bulge or are swollen, the functioning of the brain becomes dull, often leading to indecision and loss of memory.

The condition of the intestinal villi is reflected in the hair. For example, when the villi are not functioning properly as a result of being swollen and expanded, the hair will also become loose and begin to fall out. The cause in both cases is an excess of yin foods.

The Macrobiotic Approach to Digestive Diseases

1. Worms

We will consider three basic types of worms, all of which are named after their particular shapes.

A. Tapeworms. Tapeworms enter the body when we eat meat or fish that has been contaminated, and are especially common in beef and pork. Tapeworms are often present in meats that are lightly cooked, or in foods like shellfish that have spoiled. If the meat or fish is cut into thick slices, heat will often not penetrate to the central regions, and worms which are there will still be alive when it is eaten.

B. Threadworms.
1. Hookworms. This type of worm usually enters the body through the skin of the feet. From there, it travels through the bloodstream to the lungs where, through breathing, it is carried up the windpipe and swallowed into the digestive tract.
2. Pinworms. Pinworms are usually found in the large intestine, and are often discharged through the anus. They are often found on a sheet where a baby has been sleeping.

C. Whipworms. Whipworms also live in the large intestine, and their eggs are often transported in raw vegetables. It was for this reason that in the Orient, vegetables were traditionally cooked or used to make pickles, but never eaten raw. Worms of this type are more prevalent in organic vegetables, for obvious reasons.
The symptoms of worms include the following:
1. General fatigue, lack of vitality, or laziness.
2. Cravings for various foods, often accompanied by a constant feeling of hunger which is difficult to satisfy. A person with this condition will remain thin even if he consumes a large quantity of food.
3. A periodic condition of anemia.
4. An occasional feeling of nausea along with pain resembling a cramp in the area of the duodenum, which often arises several hours after the last meal.

In the Orient, this symptom is known as "worm crying."

5. Irritability, often accompanied by hysteria, screaming, and short temper. Children often exhibit this behavior when they have worms.
6. Nail-biting.
7. An indentation in the center of the thumb-nail, or a roughness in the overall condition of the nail.
8. A yellowish color in the whites of the eyes in the area closest to the nose. This is an indication of worms in about 50% of the cases in which it occurs.
9. A fragmented bowel movement.

To cure worms, it is necessary to begin the standard macrobiotic way of eating, with no raw foods. Food should be prepared with a slightly salty taste, so as to create a more alkaline condition in which worms cannot survive. Within the standard macrobiotic way of eating, the following foods are particularly advisable for the relief of this condition:

1. Raw brown rice.
2. Seeds (pumpkin, squash, watermelon, and others). These should be simply roasted without salt.
3. *Soba* (buckwheat noodles). These can be eaten daily.
4. *Mochi* (sweet brown rice).

If you suspect that you have worms, eat a handful of raw brown rice and some seeds when you become hungry. Chew each mouthful very well. As an additional symptomatic treatment, you can also drink mugwort tea. Mugwort is a wild plant that is naturally available in many areas, and in the Orient it was often mixed with *mochi*. Corsican seaweed is also helpful and can usually be obtained in oriental food stores. Boil this seaweed and drink it as a tea when you feel hungry. It can also be used in place of *bancha* tea and other beverages. As another method of curing worms, skip breakfast for several days. At lunch time, eat a large handful of raw grain combined with raw seeds like pumpkin or sunflower, and such chopped raw vegetables as scallions, garlic, and onions. At dinner, eat a normal meal. After several days, the worms will become intoxicated and begin leaving the body.

If babies or children experience itching or soreness from pinworms, mix sesame oil with grated fresh ginger (about 50% each). Apply this mixture to the itchy area with a piece of cotton and follow by applying a warm towel. If a macrobiotic baby has worms, he or she is eating too many oily, fatty, or floury foods.

2. Diseases of the Stomach

A. Stomach Ulcer. The two basic types of ulcers are those which occur in the stomach, and those found in the duodenum. In the process of digestion, the stomach secretes strong hydrochloric acid, and ulcers arise when these secretions become excessive. Mildly alkaline vegetables cause the lower stomach to secrete pepsin, and this helps to maintain a general state of balance in the condition of the stomach. However, an extremely alkaline food, such as refined sugar, stimulates the secretion of stronger acids in the upper stomach, and if this occurs constantly, the stomach lining becomes irritated and easily ruptures.

Acid-producing foods such as meat and eggs force the duodenum to accelerate its secretion of alkaline digestive juices. The over-secretion of these juices may produce an ulcer in this area. In general, ulcers which arise in the more compacted duodenum are caused by an excess of yang foods, while the overconsumption of various types of yin creates ulcers in the structurally yin stomach.

Fasting is often recommended as a way of curing ulcers. This is unnecessary, however, although proper chewing is essential. For any type of digestive disorder, including ulcers, a person should chew 200 times or more.

A person with stomach ulcers should begin the standard macrobiotic way of eating. Approximately 80% of the daily menu should consist of principal foods—whole cereal grains and cooked vegetables—while the remaining 20% can include the other supplemental foods. Among vegetables, the more compact, root vegetables should be used frequently. The standard macrobiotic way of eating is the basis for treating a duodenal ulcer. However, food should be mildly seasoned and lightly cooked. Salt should be used sparingly, and a higher percentage of leafy green or ground vegetables should be eaten. Hot applications like ginger compresses or hot salt packs are helpful for stomach ulcers, while cool applications like chlorophyll or *tofu* plasters are better for duodenal ulcers. However, ginger compresses can be effectively used for duodenal ulcers as well. In this case, apply the hot ginger compress to the stomach, and follow it with a cool compress over the area of the duodenum.

B. Stomach Cancer. Please refer to the discussion of cancer in the chapter, *The Progressive Development of Sickness.*

C. Stomach Cramps and Swelling. Stomach cramps are caused by too many yin foods, which expand the tissues and result in nerve pressure. They are similar to cramps which arise in the legs or in other parts of the body, and are caused by such excessively yin foods as soda, cold drinks, ice cream, and sugary desserts and sweets. Aside from following the standard diet, a person with this condition can obtain temporary relief by eating a handful of *gomasio*, drinking a small quantity of *umeboshi* juice, or taking *bancha* tea with several drops of *tamari*. Hot applications such as ginger compresses or roasted salt packs are also helpful,

A swollen stomach is also caused by too many expansive foods. Therefore, more compact root vegetables, like burdock and carrots, should be emphasized within the standard diet. These are particularly effective when prepared in the *kinpira* style.

3. Sicknesses of the Liver and Gall Bladder

Liver troubles often arise when this organ becomes swollen and hard and loses its functioning ability. You can diagnose this condition by trying to place your fingers under the ribcage on the right side. If you feel pain here, or are unable to place your fingers under the ribs, your liver is swollen. You should be able to insert four fingers without feeling pain.

The liver is a very important organ, so much so that in the Orient, the expression for an important occasion is *Kan-Jin* (*Kan*—liver; *Jin*—kidney). Also, in relation to the emotions, the liver was understood to govern anger. In the Orient, the term for anger is *Kan-Shaku*, meaning "liver pain." As we saw in the chapter on diagnosis, liver troubles are reflected in the face, in the area above the nose and between the eye-brows. One or more vertical lines in this area indicate liver trouble. If the lines are deep and caused by contraction, the problem is the result of too much salt and animal food. On the other hand, if the lines are caused by expansion—meaning that the skin around the lines has puffed up—the cause is too much yin.

To cure general liver troubles, which are often the result of overeating, a person can fast for several days or can eat very small quantities. Also, chewing is very important—up to 200 times per mouthful—and a person with these disorders should avoid all animal products until the condition clears up. After a brief period of fasting or semi-fasting, a person with liver problems should eat only brown rice soup with leafy green vegetables. If *miso* is added, the amount should be minimal. After several days, the range of foods can be widened to include those recommended in the standard macrobiotic way of eating, again with no animal foods, until the problem has been relieved.

External applications may be necessary if the person is experiencing pain. First apply a hot ginger compress, followed by taro potato plaster. In some cases, a person with this condition will also experience abdominal swelling due to the retention of fluid. In this case, after applying the ginger compress, apply a buckwheat plaster to the swollen region. If the person also has a fever, either a *tofu* or chlorophyll plaster can be applied to the forehead, while a small amount of *gomasio* or cooked seaweed can be eaten in cases of nausea.

A.   Jaundice.   Normally, bile secreted in the liver flows either into the gall bladder or the duodenum, where it aids in the digestive process. However, when the ducts through which bile flows become obstructed, it is then absorbed into the bloodstream. This condition, known as *jaundice*, often produces a yellowish facial and skin discoloration resulting from the accumulation of bile pigments in the skin and mucus membranes, and in some cases the urine darkens to an almost chocolate color. The primary causes of blockage in the bile ducts are foods which create fat and mucus. A person with jaundice should avoid all such foods including eggs, meat, dairy foods, sugar, oily or greasy foods, and should begin the standard macrobiotic way of eating. As with liver disorders, only vegetable quality foods should be eaten until the condition clears up, and in many cases, a fast of three to five days can be helpful. Within the range of suitable vegetables, *daikon* radish should be eaten daily in order to help dissolve these deposits. Also, mugwort tea can be used instead of other beverages until the condition improves.

Hot ginger compresses are also helpful in accelerating the melting of these deposits, and can be applied every day over the region of the liver and gall bladder until the person's condition improves. If itching develops, dip a towel into the water which you are using for the ginger compress and wash the affected area. To be effective, the water should be fairly hot.

If a nursing infant develops jaundice, the mother should eat according to the above recommendations. Once the jaundice disappears, the mother can resume the standard way of macrobiotic eating.

B.   Liver Cancer.   Please refer to the discussion of cancer in the chapter, *The Progressive Development of Sickness*.

C. Gallstones. The process leading to the formation of gallstones is similar to that for kidney stones described in the chapter, *The Progressive Development of Sickness*. Gallstones occur (1) when the bile and other bodily fluids contain plenty of sticky mucus and fatty acid, and (2) when the intake of yin, such as cold foods or beverages, crystallizes these formations into stones. In approaching this problem, we should (1) stop eating foods which contribute to the formation of mucus and fat, and (2) accelerate the dissolution and discharge of the existing stones. Within the standard macrobiotic way of eating, the selection of foods and style of preparation should be slightly yang, and vegetables such as burdock and different varieties of fall squash and pumpkins should be used often. Also, a hot ginger compress is very helpful in melting stones to a size that allows them to pass through a duct. Passing a stone can be extremely painful. In this case, immediately apply a hot ginger compress to the painful region and drink several cups of hot *bancha* tea. This will expand the duct and should allow the stone to quickly pass through.

4. Intestinal Problems

A. Appendicitis. The appendix is a relatively yang organ, since it is located in the lower part of the body and is small and tight in structure. More compacted organs are easily disturbed by an excess of yang foods, and appendicitis is caused by an excessive intake of meat, especially barbecued meats, which is an extremely yang style of preparation, as well as eggs, poultry, fish, and other similar foods. Interestingly enough, this disorder frequently occurs after a picnic or a special holiday meal, since it is often activated by alcohol and overeating. Modern medicine treats this problem by removing the appendix. This, however, usually results in a general loss of vitality and in a weakening of the legs. A person who has had his appendix removed often experiences difficulty in running or walking for extended periods.

The macrobiotic approach to appendicitis is relatively simple. In terms of diet, a person with this condition should either fast for several days or eat very simply, in a manner similar to that recommended for liver troubles. The following additional practices are useful to help relieve this condition:

1. Since appendicitis is the result of an overly yang condition caused by the consumption of too much animal food, a cool application is helpful in balancing it. A chlorophyll or tofu plaster can be used for this purpose. The chlorophyll mixture or mashed raw tofu should be about 1/2 inch in thickness, and applied so that the mixture comes in direct contact with the skin. A fresh application can be applied as soon as the mixture becomes warm.

2. It is not advisable to use the ginger compress, as the heat generated by this application could result in complications in the appendix.

3. If the person has a very high fever, apply a tofu plaster to the forehead. This can be changed every hour and a half and, as mentioned above, can also be applied to the abdomen around the area of the appendix.

If the appendix has not ruptured, an operation is unnecessary. Since it plays a crucial role in maintaining the balance of the entire intestinal region, removal of the appendix should be a last resort.

B. Enteritis (Inflammation of the Intestinal Tract). Symptoms such as diarrhea, constipation, abdominal pain, and fever are often associated with this condition. Enteritis can be either chronic or acute, and both can be caused by extremes of either yin or yang foods.

In the acute type, a person will experience pain which may be accompanied by diarrhea or fever. If this condition results from the intake of some extremely yin food, hot applications such as ginger compresses or roasted salt can be used for relief. Of course, the person should also stop the intake of all extreme foods, and maintain the standard diet. If, on the other hand, the condition is caused by too many yang foods, a taro potato plaster or other cool application should be used, and the person should temporarily eliminate all animal products.

Chronic enteritis develops slowly and is caused by the repeated consumption of overly-yin or overly-yang foods. Many people suffer from this condition—possibly more than 75% of the population of the United States. The most common symptom is the lack of a smooth, healthy bowel movement. Instead, persons with this condition have a very irregular bowel movement—sometimes they are constipated and sometimes they have diarrhea. This condition can be diagnosed in the face by a swollen lower lip. If you observe the photographs of fashion models on the covers of magazines, or notice the lower lips of people in general, you will begin to realize just how widespread this problem is.

To relieve these chronic intestinal problems, we should begin eating according to the general macrobiotic standard. This will help the intestine to regain its normal elasticity and functioning ability. Persons with chronic intestinal disorders should limit their intake of bread and other flour products, nut butters and other oily or greasy foods, as well as fruit juice and other very yin items. Foods like *miso* and *tamari*, which contain living bacteria beneficial to digestion and assimilation, should be eaten daily in soup. Other processed or fermented foods such as pickles and *umeboshi* plums also help to strengthen the intestines. Of course, proper chewing is essential in curing any type of intestinal troubles.

1. Dysentery. Dysentery can be caused by amoebae, worms, bacteria, or chemical poisons which irritate the intestines. This ailment frequently occurs during travel in an area where the food or water is unclean. Dysentery is often characterized by diarrhea, cramps, pain in the abdomen, and sometimes mucus or blood in the stools. This condition is often chronic, and may last several months.

Within the standard macrobiotic diet, the best item for relieving this condition is the *umeboshi* plum, or the juice which is extracted from it. If you plan to travel extensively in a place such as India, Africa, or South America, take a large supply of *umeboshi* plums with you, enough so that you can eat one or two every morning along with some *bancha* tea. *Umeboshi* is very effective in neutralizing harmful bacteria, and will help prevent both dysentery and cholera. However, if you do get dysentery, mix *umeboshi* juice in *bancha* tea and drink this every couple of hours. If *umeboshi* plums are not available, add salt to cooked rice or other whole grain and chew it thoroughly. Avoid all salad, fruits, or raw foods until your condition improves, and minimize your liquid intake. If you are still in one of these countries, boil all of the water that you use for drinking or cooking. When your condition improves, return to the standard way of macrobiotic eating.

2. Cholera. The symptoms of cholera include high fever, diarrhea, vomiting, and in some cases, an inability to walk. The dietary approach to this problem is the same as for dysentery. A *tofu* or chlorophyll plaster can be applied to the head to relieve a fever, and to strengthen the intestines, apply a roasted salt pack to the abdomen. If the person is nauseous or is vomiting frequently, have him drink *umeboshi* juice with some grated ginger, while a hot hip bath is helpful in cases of leg cramps. Dried *daikon*, turnip or other green leaves and mustard powder should be added to the hot bath water, but if these are not available, salt can be substituted. This will improve circulation in the lower part of the body. If there is no place to take a hot bath, apply a ginger compress, mustard plaster, or hot water compress to the abdomen or other painful areas.

   3. Echerichia (Children's Dysentery).   This condition can be prevented by avoiding peaches, apples, bananas, and other tree fruits. However, strawberries and other more yang fruits that grow on the ground usually will not cause this problem caused by excess yin. Children who develop this condition should avoid raw vegetables and fruits until it disappears completely. The basic dietary approach for this illness is the same as for the above conditions, and again, *tofu* or chlorophyll plasters can be applied to the head for the relief of fever. Rather than a hot hip bath (which can be difficult for children), apply hot towels to the painful regions. After their condition improves, they can return to the standard macrobiotic way of eating. Since children require much less salt than adults, when treating this condition with *umeboshi* juice or salt, be careful not to use too much.

C.   Colitis.   This is an inflammation of the large intestine, frequently accompanied by excessive secretions of mucus. For relief, begin the standard macrobiotic way of eating and apply hot compresses over the intestinal region. Hot *tamari-bancha* is also helpful. Colitis can be the result of the overconsumption of either extremely yin or yang foods which produce an acidic blood and body condition.

D.   Hernia.   A hernia arises when the wall of the stomach or intestines becomes loose, expands, and descends. An operation is the standard method of treatment, but this does not eliminate the cause or change the over-expanded condition of the organs and tissues. The normal contracted state of tissues and organs can be re-established only through proper diet. A hernia can usually be relieved in four to six months with the standard macrobiotic approach, including the following practices:
   1.   Watercress, kale, leeks, cabbage, *daikon* and carrot greens, and other tough, fibrous vegetables should be eaten often to strengthen the muscles of the intestinal walls.
   2.   A side dish of *hijiki* seaweed, which contains plenty of minerals, should be eaten every day.
   3.   Salt is required to cause contraction of the intestinal or stomach tissues. Unrefined sea salt should be used for this purpose in cooking, along with high-quality vegetable oil.
   4.   Persons who are overweight should try to return to their normal weight.
   5.   All yin foods such as ice cream, fruit, sugar, excess liquid, and others should be avoided. As little as half an orange can cause the intestinal tissues to become loose and expanded.

6. Long, hot baths and showers should be avoided, because they take minerals out of the body.
7. In cases where the intestinal tissue begins to protrude, a hot, steaming towel can be applied to the anus, followed by an application of sesame oil. Then, push the protruding tissue back with your finger.
8. A support should be worn, and plenty of physical activity is recommended.

Persons with this condition can return to the standard macrobiotic way of eating after the hernia disappears. This will prevent a recurrence.

E. Hemorrhoids. Hemorrhoids arise from two basic causes: (1) the overconsumption of various types of yin food which cause the blood capillaries in the rectum to expand and rupture, and (2) the overconsumption of foods such as eggs, meat, and fish, which cause the tissues to contract and bleed. To relieve yin hemorrhoids, begin the standard diet and avoid fruit, salad, excessive liquid and other expansive foods. For yang hemorrhoids, avoid all animal products, while keeping the intake of salt to a minimum. In both cases, return to the standard way of eating after the condition improves.

Appendix

The Effects of Sugar

In regard to refined sugar, we need to consider the different effects produced in the body by the three main varieties of sugar: simple sugars or *monosaccharides*, which are found in fruits and honey; double sugars or *disaccharides*, which are found in cane sugar and milk; and complex sugars or *polysaccharides*, which are found in grains, beans, and vegetables.

In the normal digestive process, grain sugars, or polysaccharides, are first decomposed by saliva in the mouth, then further broken down in the stomach, and then completely digested in the duodenum and intestines.

When refined sugar enters the stomach, it causes what is known as a "sugar reaction," whereby the stomach is temporarily paralyzed. As little as 1/4 teaspoon of refined sugar can cause this. Since refined sugar is strongly alkaloid, the stomach secretes unusual amounts of acid in order to make balance, which, if repeated over a long enough period, can cause eventual ulceration of the stomach wall. Our blood normally maintains a weak alkaline condition, and when strongly alkaline refined sugar is introduced, what is known as an "acid reaction" takes place, causing the bloodstream to become over-acidic. To compensate for this, our internal supply of minerals is mobilized so as to restore a more normal balance. The minerals in our daily food and in our normal body reserve are sufficient to meet this situation if it arises now and then. However, if we are eating refined sugar every day, this supply is not sufficient, and we must depend on minerals stored deep within the body, particularly calcium in our bones and teeth. If this continues for a long enough period, the depletion of calcium from the bones and teeth results in their eventual decay and general weakening.

Excess sugar is stored in various places within the body, first in the form of *gly-*

cogen in the liver. When the amount of glycogen exceeds the liver's storage capacity of about 50 grams, it is then released into the bloodstream in the form of fatty acid, which is first stored in the more inactive places of the body such as the buttocks, thighs, and mid-section. Then, if the intake of refined sugar is continued, this fatty acid becomes attracted to the more active organs such as the heart and kidneys, which gradually become encased in a layer of fat and mucus, which also penetrate the inner tissues of these organs. This of course weakens their normal functioning, and when excessive enough causes their eventual stoppage. The growing consumption of refined sugar in modern nations can be seen in the increasing incidence of such degenerative diseases as heart disease, which two out of five people in the United States are now suffering from. Refined sugar also directly affects our thinking abilities, through the destruction of the intestinal bacteria which are responsible for the creation of B-Vitamins necessary for the synthesis of glutamic acid which is directly involved in the mental activities carried on in the brain. A lack of this component can result in a lack of memory and ability to think clearly.

In general, the intake of refined sugar, which is a highly processed and refined product of tropical climates, results in an overall yinnization of our physical and mental condition, particularly affecting the parasympathetic nervous system, and the organs which it governs. This is what cases "sugar reaction" in the stomach mentioned earlier. Sweeteners such as honey and maple syrup have an effect similar to that of refined sugar, although to a lesser degree, and should be avoided as much as possible in daily use.*

---

* For additional information regarding the physiological and psychological effects of refined sugar, please see *Sugar Blues* by William Dufty, published by Chilton Book Company, 1975.

CHAPTER FIVE

The Respiratory System

The purpose of respiration in man and animals is to provide the body's cells with oxygen and to facilitate the discharge of carbon dioxide. The two types of respiration are (1) internal respiration, which entails the exchange of oxygen and carbon dioxide between the tissue cells and their surrounding fluid, and (2) external respiration, in which the body exchanges these gases with the surrounding atmosphere. Being yang, animals are attracted to oxygen, which is yin, and repel the more yang carbon dioxide. The major components of the human respiratory system include (1) the nasal passages and the sinuses; (2) the larynx and vocal cords; (3) the trachea or windpipe, which is located in front of the esophagus; (4) the bronchi and bronchioli; (5) the alveoli, or air sacs; and (6) the lungs.

The lungs are asymmetrical, as are all the paired organs of the body. (See Fig. 38.) The left lung is composed of two lobes, and the right lung has three. Two bronchial arteries go to the left lung, and one to the right. These arteries follow the bronchi, and their branches supply nourishment to the lung tissues. Bronchial veins run along these branches in the opposite direction.

De-oxygenated blood enters the lungs through the pulmonary arteries, which come from the right side of the heart. The branches of this artery end in a net of capillaries which surround each of the alveoli. After blood has been supplied with oxygen, it is collected in the pulmonary veins, which transport it to the left auricle of the heart for distribution to all of the body's tissues. The lungs are surrounded by the *thoracic*, or *pleural cavity*, which is lined by a thin, moist membrane called the *pleura*.

The Macrobiotic Approach to Respiratory Diseases

1. Emphysema

Emphysema was virtually unknown before the Second World War. Since then, the number of people afflcted with this disease has grown logarithmically. The widespread increase of this yin sickness parallels the postwar proliferation of artificially-produced, chemicalized food, such as ice cream and soft drinks, frozen fruit juice, and others.

The overconsumption of these excessive foods causes the alveoli to dilate and fuse, so that the lung tissue as a whole becomes loose. Within the lung, the surface area used for the exchange of oxygen and carbon dioxide diminishes, and a person compensates for this by breathing more rapidly. Emphysema generally results in death from an overworked heart. Dilation of the bronchi can be remedied with more yang food and saltier cooking. However, once the alveoli have started to fuse, it is very difficult to separate them. If the blood becomes thicker, the fused sacs may shrink but in most cases will not separate. The standard macrobiotic way of eating can stop the development of the disease, however.

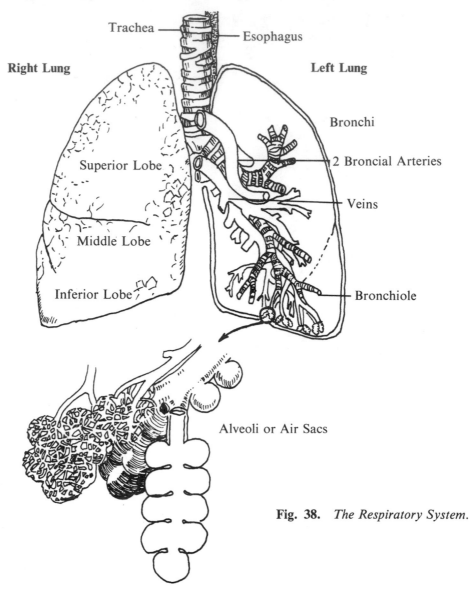

Fig. 38. *The Respiratory System.*

2. Lung Mucus

Deep, wheezing breaths occur when the walls of the bronchi are covered with mucus. This is caused by foods such as dairy products, sugar, fruits, and saturated fats. The mechanism whereby this condition develops is discussed in the chapter, *The Progressive Development of Sickness*. In more serious cases, mucus begins to fill the alveoli, and breathing becomes difficult. Occasionally, a coat of mucus may even develop around the air sacs, choking off the blood supply. Mucus in the bronchi can be loosened and discharged by coughing, but once it surrounds the sacs, it becomes more firmly lodged, and may remain there for years. Then, if air pollutants and cigarette smoke enter the lungs, their more solid components are attracted to and remain in this sticky environment. In severe cases, these deposits can trigger the development of lung cancer. However, air pollution or cigarette smoke are not the causes of this disease. The real problem lies in the condition of the alveoli and the blood and capillaries which surround them.

Recently, a remote village was studied in South America, where the natives begin smoking at about the age of five, and continue throughout life, with no evidence of lung disease. Unlimited heavy smoking is, of course, not advisable, but neither is breathing heavily polluted air. The real cause of these problems is poor quality blood, resulting from improper diet, and the most fundamental way of preventing them and treating them is proper eating.

3.   Asthma

Asthma is characterized by constant coughing and difficult or labored breathing, which often leads to a violent attack. This is caused by an obstruction of the respiratory passages, either by a spasm of the muscles in the bronchial tubes, or by the secretion of excessive amounts of mucus. Since asthma is more prevalent in wet climates, a drier environment is usually healthier for persons with this yin condition.

The best approach for asthma is to begin the standard macrobiotic way of eating, while limiting the intake of liquid, including the amount of water used in cooking. Of course, the consumption of other forms of yin, such as fruit and salad, should also be reduced. With this method, it is possible to relieve asthma within several weeks. Interestingly enough, asthma is often associated with many years of overworking the kidneys, resulting from the repeated overconsumption of fluid.

Asthma is presently treated with very strong medications which cause the bronchial tubes to dilate, thus making breathing easier. However, since asthma is caused by excess yin, this treatment will actually aggravate the condition. To cure asthma, we need to produce a contraction or tightening of the bronchial tubes, which can be accomplished only through the appropriate way of eating.

If a person with asthma feels an attack coming on, a hot ginger compress applied repeatedly to the upper chest will help lessen its severity. At the same time, the person should eat a small handful of *gomasio* or several *umeboshi* plums, which will cause the alveoli to immediately contract. These can be easily carried with you in case of an attack outside the home.

4.   Bronchitis and Pneumonia

In order to understand these conditions, let us consider the similarity between the respiratory system and a tree. (See Fig. 39.)

In many ways, the lungs resemble an inverted tree. The roots and stem of a tree are compacted, and the leaves are more expanded. The leaves, being yin, attract carbon dioxide and repel oxygen. In the lungs, this is reversed; the trachea, which corresponds to the tree stem, is hollow, while the alveoli, which correspond to the leaves, are more compacted. Since the alveoli are yang, they attract oxygen and discharge carbon dioxide.

Bronchitis is a disease of the trachea and bronchi, the yin section of the lungs. When the sickness is deeper—involving the alveoli—it is called pneumonia. Persons with a more frail constitution would tend to develop bronchitis, while a person who

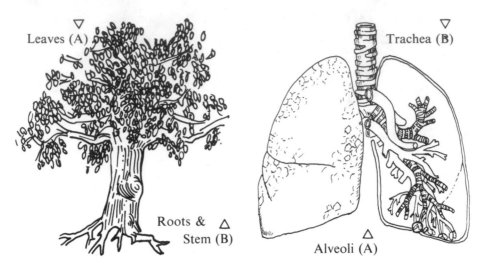

Fig. 39. *The leaves of the tree (A) correspond to the alveoli or air sacs (A), while the roots and stem (B) correspond to the trachea (B).*

is stronger, more sturdy, and often a big meat-eater is more frequently afflicted with pneumonia. Bronchitis has a yin character—lingering for a long time—while pneumonia is the opposite: it usually develops abruptly and is more acute.

A. Bronchitis. Bronchitis is generally accompanied by coughing and chest pain, and many "colds" are actually a mild form of it. As we have seen, bronchitis is a yin sickness, since (1) it is longer-lasting and takes more time to cure; (2) it tends to develop in the autumn; (3) the primary method of discharge is through coughing; and (4) the fever associated with it is usually mild.

The overconsumption of foods like cold drinks, fruit, ice cream, and sugar is the cause of bronchitis. Naturally, to relieve this condition, we should eliminate these items and begin the standard macrobiotic way of eating. The fever that accompanies bronchitis is usually beneficial, since it represents the body's attempt to discharge or burn off excess. However, if the fever becomes dangerously high, it should be reduced by applying a *tofu* or chlorophyll plaster to the forehead. While these symptoms occur, the patient should eat only hot foods. Also, hot applications like the ginger compress or mustard plaster should be applied regularly to the chest for relief.

B. Pneumonia. Pneumonia is a more yang type of sickness, since (1) it develops suddenly, and if it is not properly treated, can result in death within several days; (2) it arises more during the spring and summer; (3) the coughing accompanying it is less frequent than with bronchitis; and (4) it produces a high, burning fever. When a person dies of this disease, it is because the lobes of the lungs have become clogged, putting an unbearable strain on the heart.

Pneumonia is caused by the repeated consumption of extremes such as meat, eggs, and other animal products. However, although the underlying cause is yang, the symptoms are activated by yin, in the form of fruit juice, cold drinks, sugar, and other items. For this reason, people who don't consume meat usually do not develop pneumonia. A person with this condition should immediately stop eating all of these foods and begin the standard diet. The recommended applications given above can also be very helpful.

The modern medical approach to this disease is usually effective in relieving the accompanying symptoms. However, since it does not consider or attempt to remedy the cause of the problem, it should not be thought of as a cure. Along with suggesting the necessary modifications in a patient's diet, traditional practitioners of oriental medicine treated the symptoms of pneumonia by placing cold applications over the lungs. The most effective of these is a carp plaster. Carp is a very yin fish, and has been found effective in neutralizing the fever and overly-yang condition associated with pneumonia.

If you can obtain a live carp, first offer your thanks and appreciation to it, and, after killing it, extract a small quantity of its blood. This should be taken in a small cup, about the size of a *saké* cup. Infants should drink 1/8 of a cup; children should have 1/4; and adults should take 1/2 cup. This will help t reduce the fever. Meanwhile, wrap the carp in a towel and crush it with a hammer in the same way you would crush a piece of ice. Apply this to the chest, and check the person's temperature every half hour, since it will drop quickly. Remove the application when the temperature drops to 97 degrees. This may take from one to three hours, or longer in some cases. It may even be necessary to apply a fresh plaster, but the temperature will eventually drop and breathing will become easier. This is one of the most effective methods for relieving the symptoms of pneumonia, even in advanced cases.

If carp is unavailable, you can apply a *tofu*, chlorophyll, or potato plaster, and even ice or cold ground beef can be helpful. Since this type of meat contains plenty of fat, it is effective for reducing a fever, although it is not recommended for eating.

Since the symptoms of bronchitis and pneumonia are often similar, we must accurately determine from which the person is suffering. If our judgment is faulty, and we apply the wrong treatment, the person could die.

5. Tuberculosis

In medical terms, tuberculosis is an infectious disease caused by an acid bacteria, *Mycobacterium tuberculosis*. This particular type of bacteria is relatively weak, since this disease develops over a comparatively long time, and the bacterium is easily killed by sunlight. Tuberculosis can arise in the bones and joints, kidneys, bladder, intestines, lymph glands, or in any part of the body, but the most common form develops in the lungs. At one time, tuberculosis was the leading cause of death in the United States.

In the primary, or first infection stage, known also as *childhood tuberculosis*, the lymph nodes in the central part of the lung, around the entrance to the bronchi, become enlarged and calcified. In this stage, the disease is considered to be non-infectious. The secondary, or reinfection type, known also as *adult tuberculosis*, is characterized by the formation of cavities in the lungs. The walls of these cavities gradually calcify and increase in size, and as a result, the inner lung tissue gradually decomposes. At this stage, the disease is actively infectious, since the many bacteria which inhabit the lung cavities are often transmitted through breathing.

The medical treatment of this disease has varied. At one time a diet rich in animal foods was recommended. This approach was later changed, and sun baths were considered best. As we have seen, tuberculosis is a yin disease and the bacteria are easily killed by sunlight. As this disease develops, the blood vessels within the lungs become weak and rupture, and blood is often coughed up. This condition is often aggravated by sunlight, which stimulates blood circulation. For this reason, it is better for someone with this disease to stay inside and perform only light physical activity.

A later treatment involved puncturing the skin and forcefully injecting air into the cavity between the rib cage and the lungs. Another approach, known as *thoracoplasty*, involves removing a portion of the ribs in order to alter the shape of the lung. The most recent method of treating tuberculosis is to administer antibiotics over a long period of time. Meanwhile, if the patient's condition is infectious, he must be isolated in a sanatorium where his condition is monitored. If, after several tests, it is determined that he is no longer emitting bacteria, he is pronounced "clean" and discharged.

In order to cure tuberculosis, we must first understand its cause. Tuberculosis develops as a result of the repeated consumpton of both extremely yin and extremely yang foods. As we have seen in the chapter, *The Progressive Development of Sickness*, the repeated intake of extremes such as meat and sugar creates a strong acid condition in the blood which elicits a buffer reaction that draws on the body's reserve of minerals. Calcium comprises 40% of the body's mineral content, and is the element used most often in this process. If we have a daily minor acidosis, the buffer maintains the necessary alkaline condition in our body, and the effects are not usually serious. However, when the intake of excess exceeds the bloodstream's capacity to neutralize it, deposits of fatty acid and mucus begin to accumulate in the lungs, kidneys, lymph nodes, and other places. In an attempt to neutralize these additional acidic deposits, buffer reactions begin to take place around the site of the localization. As a result, various regions of the particular organ begin to calcify, and bacteria thrive in this highly acidic environment. This condition is known as tuberculosis.

To relieve this condition, we need to stop the intake of sugar, fruit, meat, dairy products, soft drinks, eggs, fish, refined grains, and other extreme foods which produce an acidic condition. A person with tuberculosis should begin the standard macrobiotic way of eating, with emphasis on well-cooked root vegetables like carrots and burdock. The cooking should be strong and fairly salty. A person with this condition should also control the intake of liquid.

6. Whooping Cough

In the Orient, the name for this disease is "100 days' cough," since it usually continues for about that length of time. Whooping cough is related to the symptoms of discharge which arise during the course of a season, or "100 days."

The effects of the food we eat remain in the body for about three months, since the red blood cells, which are synthesized from food, have a life span of about 120 days. To illustrate how whooping cough develops, suppose a person eats an extreme food, like ice cream or tomatoes, in early March. Since this is a more yin time of year, an imbalance is created, and this excess takes about 120 days to be totally expelled. Whooping cough arises when this excess is discharged through the lungs in the form of coughing. As the season changes to summer, a time span corresponding approximately to the period that the excess remains in the body, the discharge is completed and the illness disappears. However, it is not necessary to wait 100 days for this to happen. By eating more strongly-cooked foods, this internal imbalance can be neutralized within several weeks. Persons with this condition should begin the standard way of eating with a slight emphasis toward a yang selection of foods and style of preparation.

7. Hay Fever (Allergic Reactions)

Hay fever is usually accompanied by sneezing, a runny nose, and in some cases, fever. It is widely believed that an allergy to pollen causes this condition. However, pollen is not the cause of hay fever. If it were, then everyone would develop it. Why is it that some people react this way, some mildly, and others more severely, while others are not affected at all? The primary cause of this susceptibility to irritation is the consumption of dairy food, and especially cold milk; while fruit, chemicals, sugar, and other forms of yin also contribute to this condition.

Since pollen is yin, when it enters the body a reaction occurs: like repels like, resulting in draining, sneezing, and coughing. This arises only when the condition of the blood is not good, when it contains too much yin. These foods also make the condition of the blood and internal mucus membranes sticky, and when pollen is inhaled, it sticks and produces irritation rather than being smoothly discharged, Hay fever and other chronic allergies can be easily relieved through the standard macrobiotic way of eating.

8. Pleurisy

Pleurisy is a pooling of water in the area between the rib cage and the membranes which cover the lungs. With this condition, deep breathing is accompanied by pressure and pain, and if it continues beyond several days, a fever of between 100 and 103 degrees often develops. Pleurisy usually lasts between one and three months, during which time the patient is advised to rest in bed.

This condition is simply the result of an excessive intake of liquid, especially cold or iced beverages and products like frozen fruit juices. Watery foods also contribute to this condition, as does sugar and ther items which rapidly dissolve into water after being eaten. This problem can be relieved in one week through the standard macrobiotic approach. As with asthma, our aim is to make the person's condition less watery by serving drier foods and by limiting the intake of liquid. The discharge of excess fluid can be accelerated by the application of hot ginger compresses to the lung region.

Appendix

The Voice

Speech depends on the following basic factors: (1) outgoing breath; (2) a vibrator, or the vocal cords; (3) an amplifier, or the pharynx, mouth, and nasal cavity; and

(4) the lips, tongue, the hard and soft palates, the walls of the mouth, and the nasal cavities, all of which act as articulators.

Before puberty, boys and girls have the same general voice pitch. At the time of puberty, however, a boy's voice becomes deeper, while a girl's generally stays the same. This transitory period lasts for about two years, after which a boy's voice becomes noticeably lower and masculine. Boys become more yang at the time of puberty, and this causes excess to be released into the bloodstream. This is often discharged through physical activity, but some of it is attracted to the vocal cords, causing them to expand and the voice to lower. Girls don't experience this condition since their excess is more efficiently discharged through menstruation.

Let us consider the following difficulties which arise with speech and respiration, along with several related problems:

1. Stuttering. Stuttering is often caused by the overconsumption of foods which expand the vocal cords and inhibit their ability to vibrate. This condition can gradually be improved through proper eating.

2. Inability to Speak Due to Brain Malfunction. This can occur when either the motor center or sensory center of the brain begins to malfunction. Excessive yin causes the motor center to malfunction, while excess yang causes problems in the sensory center. This condition takes several months to cure, during which time the person should observe the standard macrobiotic diet, with emphasis on proper chewing.

3. Hiccoughing. This occurs when the diaphragm becomes loose, as a result of an excess of yin foods, and begins to repeatedly contract. Take a small handful of *gomasio* every 15 minutes to relieve this problem. *Tekka*, sea salt, or *umeboshi* are also useful.

4. Snoring. Snoring is caused by excess yin, and especially by the overconsumption of liquids. Items such as milk, fruit juice, alcohol, and coffee expand and loosen the uvula, causing it to vibrate excessively. They also contribute to the development of mucus in the nose and sinus cavities, which can obstruct breathing through the nasal passages. Snoring can be cured very quickly by controlling the liquid intake.

5. Bad Breath (Halitosis). Bad breath originating in the lungs indicates that the quality of the blood has become poor. Foods such as animal protein, saturated fat, and sugar cause the blood to become acidic, and to have an unpleasant odor. This condition can be cured by eating very well for several weeks. If bad breath comes from the stomach, it is caused by the decomposition of food. This more temporary condition can be quickly relieved by taking *umeboshi*, *tamari-bancha*, or grated *daikon*.

6. Belching. Belching is caused by eating in a disorderly way. The yang foods in our meal should be eaten first, followed by the more yin items. For example, if our meal consists of 50% grains with two side dishes of vegetables, we should begin with the grain and alternate with the more yang vegetable dish until it is finished. Then, we should proceed to alternate the remaining grain with the more yin vegetable until the meal is completed. If we do not follow this order in our eating, the secretion of stomach juices becomes unbalanced and belching often results.

CHAPTER SIX

The Circulatory and Lymphatic Systems

The Blood

Our blood is a replica of the ancient sea in which biological life developed for seven-eighths of its long evolutionary history. At first this water was fresh or clear, but as minerals were leeched from the earth, it became increasingly salty. Biological life has existed on earth for about 3.2 billion years. For approximately the first 2.8 billion years, evolution took place in water, while about 400 million years were spent on land.

During the nine months of pregnancy, we repeat the evolutionary process of life in water. We grow in a liquid environment during the embryonic period, and in this sense are very much like fish. At birth, contractions force us out of the womb, and we become air-breathing land animals. These birth contractions correlate to the alternating rising and sinking of land that occurred on earth about 400 million years ago. Our salty bloodstream replicates the saline ocean environment from which life emerged and our lymph liquid and urine also reflect this heritage.

The blood consists of liquid in the form of plasma and *formed elements*, which are the more yang red and more yin white cells and the blood platelets. The plasma comprises about 55% of the blood by volume, while the various formed elements, which are suspended in the plasma, constitute the remaining 45%.

1.   Red Blood Cells (Erythrocytes)

Our bodies contain about 35 trillion red blood cells. (See Fig. 40.) Each of these tiny disc-shaped cells is about 7.7 microns in diameter and about 1.9 microns thick. Men have about 5 million per cubic mm, and women about 4.5 million per cubic mm. The number of red blood cells is dependent on a variety of circumstances. For example, as we grow older, their number decreases from the six million per cubic mm that we had at birth. This is one reason why newborn infants and babies are very yang. Also, the number of red blood cells increases as the altitude at which we live increases. People living at elevations of 10,000 feet or more above sea level are generally more yang than those living at lower altitudes. Their red blood cell counts are as much as 30 per cent above normal. When we are in a more active state, the number of red blood cells increases, while during sleep, the number decreases. The number of red cells also multiplies as muscular activity or environmental temperature rises.

Hemoglobin comprises between 60 and 80 per cent of the red blood cell. This percentage varies between men and women. Men have about 16 grams per 100 cc of blood, and women about 14 grams per 100 cc. Hemoglobin consists of *hematin*, which is a more yang form of protein containing iron, as well as a simpler yin protein. Hematin attracts oxygen in the lungs and transports it to the cells. Then, as

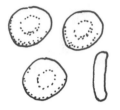

Fig. 40. *Red blood cells (erythrocytes) comprise a more yang component of the blood stream. Front and side views shown.*

the oxygen-depleted blood returns through the veins, it attracts and transports carbon dioxide back to the lungs where it is exhaled. This process is essential for life and the efficiency with which it is accomplished directly influences our health. (See Fig. 41.) In a normal adult, about 20 million red blood cells are destroyed every minute. New red blood cells are continuously formed to replace them. The total volume of hemoglobin in the body is about one kilogram, 20 grams of which are destroyed and rebuilt every day.

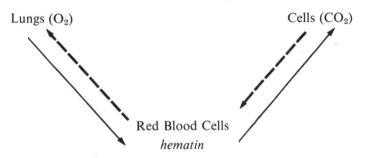

Fig. 41. *In the lungs, the hematin portion of the red blood cells attracts and combines with oxygen, which is then transported to the cells. Hemoglobin also carries carbon dioxide back to the lungs where it is exhaled.*

2. White Blood Cells (Leucocytes)

The human body contains far fewer white than red blood cells—about 6,000 per cubic mm. (See Fig. 42.) They are usually larger than red blood cells, possess a nucleus, and have the power of movement similar to that of an amoeba. White blood cells are attracted to bacteria entering the body, which they envelop and devour. They also gather around inflamed external injuries. White blood cells are divided into two general groups: *granulocytes* and *agranulocytes*. Granulocytes are subdivided into three types: *neutrophils, eosinophils,* and *basophils*, while agranulocytes are subdivided into *lymphocytes* and *monocytes*.

The Macrobiotic Approach to Blood Diseases

1. Leukemia

In this disease, the number of red blood cells decreases while the number of white blood cells increases dramatically. In some cases, leukemia patients may have as many as one million white blood cells per cubic mm instead of the normal 5,000–

GRANULOCYTES

9–12 microns

Neutrophilis
3–5 lobes in nucleus

9–12 microns

Eosinophilis
2 lobes in nucleus

18 microns

Basophilis
Indistinctly lobed nucleus

AGRANULOCYTES

8–12 microns

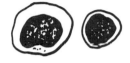

Lymphocytes

12–15 microns

Monocytes

Fig. 42. *The varieties of white blood cells, all of which are more yin than red blood cells.*

6,000. Leukemia can be either chronic or acute, and there is no medical cure for this illness which often results in death. Leukemia is relatively easy to control, however, through proper eating.

White blood cells are yin. An increase in their number indicates an overconsumption of extreme foods, especially sugar, soft drinks, ice cream, milk, and chemicals. At the same time, a decrease in the number of red blood cells reflects a lack of minerals and other high-quality yang foods in the diet. The mechanism by which this condition develops is discussed in the chapter, *The Progressive Development of Sickness*, page 29, while a more comprehensive list of the foods causing leukemia, which is a more yin type of cancer, is found in the same chapter. The dietary recommendations for the relief of this condition are similar to those for the relief of other yin cancers, and are listed on page 44. As with other types of cancer, a person with leukemia should chew up to 150 or 200 times per mouthful. However, in cases where the quality of the person's saliva is not good, a healthier person should chew the food and then spoon-feed the patient.

A hot ginger compress can also be applied daily to the *hara* region. This will stimulate the normal production of healthy red blood cells by the intestinal villi. With this approach, leukemia can be reversed in a relatively short time.

2. Anemia

Anemia is a deficiency of red blood cells, hemoglobin, or total blood volume. The symptoms of anemia include (1) gray or white lips (the lips should be pink); (2) a white color in the inside of the lower eyelid (this should also be pink); (3) pale or white cheeks; (4) white rather than pink fingernails; (5) a lack of vitality; and (6) a decrease in sexual activity. The three main types of this illness are nutritional anemia, pernicious anemia, and sickle-cell anemia.

A. Nutritional Anemia. Nutritional anemia results from a deficiency of various substances which are necessary in the production of red blood cells, such as iron, cobalt, copper, various proteins, and vitamins such as B-12 and folic acid. Persons with this condition are usually advised by doctors to take iron or vitamin supplements or to eat large quantities of meat. This approach may temporarily relieve symptoms, but it ignores the underlying cause of anemia. If we have a good balance of yin and yang in our daily food and activity, we synthesize our own iron without having to rely on artificial measures. This synthesis occurs in the body through the natural process of transmutation.

Iron is the core of hemoglobin, which is the basis of animal life. The basis of plant life is chlorophyll, the center of which is magnesium. (See Fig. 43.) Since their peripheral elements are the same, the difference between chlorophyll and hemoglobin lies in the magnesium and iron which comprise their respective centers. All animals eat vegetables which contain chlorophyll, either directly or indirectly, and use it to create hemoglobin. Since the peripheral elements are the same for both, magnesium must be changing into iron within the bodies of animals, including man. This transmutation occurs with the addition of two atoms of oxygen, and is symbolized in the following formula:

$$\substack{12\\24}Mg + \substack{16\\32}O_2 \longrightarrow \substack{26\\56}Fe(Co, Ni)$$

Nutritional anemia results primarily from a lack of chlorophyll in the diet as well as the overconsumption of yin foods which hinder the normal production of red blood cells. A fundamental cure can be achieved through the standard macrobiotic way of eating, with particular emphasis on green leafy vegetables like kale, *daikon* leaves, watercress, and others which contain large amounts of chlorophyll. Beans and fermented soybean products which contain high-quality protein are also beneficial because they increase vitality. A person with this type of anemia should keep physically active, so as to increase his intake of oxygen. At the same time, hot ginger compresses can be applied to the small intestine in order to stimulate the production of healthy red blood cells.

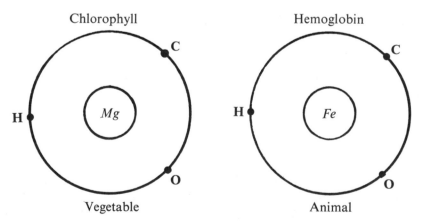

Fig. 43. *In the human body, chlorophyll changes into hemoglobin through a process of transmutation in which magnesium changes into iron. This is accomplished with the addition of oxygen.*

B. Pernicious Anemia. In pernicious anemia, the red blood cells increase in size while decreasing in number. The symptoms of this illness include pallor, weakness, and gastrointestinal and nervous disturbances, all of which are associated with a lack of gastric juice containing what is called an intrinsic factor. Pernicious anemia is believed to result from a lack of Vitamin B-12, which is sometimes referred to as the "anti-pernicious anemia vitamin." A lack of this vitamin results in retarded growth and a high rate of mortality in offspring. Many people believe that Vitamin B-12 is available only in foods of animal origin like milk, organ meat, and egg yolks.

However, for centuries, millions of people have lived without many animal products, and yet did not develop pernicious anemia. Vitamin B-12 is found in the milk and liver of cows. These animals subsist entirely on grasses which do not contain B-12. Apparently they have the ability to synthesize the vitamin within their own digestive tracts. It would seem logical that, as more highly developed animals, humans should also have this ability. Since recent nutritional studies have shown that Vitamin B-12 exists in fermented vegetable foods like *miso* and *tamari*, as well as in some seaweeds, if pernicious anemia arises, it is not necessary to eat animal products. Also, this illness may develop as a result of our losing our natural ability to synthesize Vitamin B-12, and it may be possible to recover this ability once we stop eating animal foods. Persons with pernicious anemia should observe the standard macrobiotic way of eating, with a bowl of *miso* soup every day. Seaweeds should also be eaten on a regular basis.

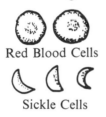

Red Blood Cells

Sickle Cells

Fig. 44. *The transformation of red blood cells into sickle cells.*

C. Sickle-Cell Anemia. (See Fig. 44.) This disease is a special problem in the United States. About 10% of the Negro population in America are so-called "carriers." This amounts to between two and three million people. Among this group, one out of about every 400 becomes seriously ill or dies from the illness. This disease usually occurs before the age of 20, and develops almost exclusively within the Negro population. The main symptoms are periodic attacks of paralysis similar to epilepsy, fatigue, and brain damage. A person with this condition often starts to forget simple things and will frequently experience pain in the nerves or muscles. In severe cases, the person curls up in the embryo position and cannot move. Sickle-cell anemia often results in death, and there is no medical cure for it.

The most prevalent theory about the cause of sickle-cell anemia states that Negroes, who originally lived in malaria-infested West Africa, carry an anti-malaria factor in their blood. Purportedly, this factor is created by the transformation of red blood cells into sickle cells. This condition is considered hereditary and appears in black people in both Africa and the United States. Scientists assert that as long as they remain in Africa—where malaria is common—there is no trouble, because of the yang climate and the natural diet. Once black people move to another climate, however, with different environmental factors, this condition becomes a threat to their lives.

There is another theory, however, which states that sickle-cell anemia has only recently become widespread, probably only since the end of World War II. The consumption of refined, processed foods like sugar, soft drinks, ice cream, refined flour, and chemicals, has contributed to this condition. Red blood cells are yang, while sickle cells are yin. The increased incidence of this disease coincides with the increase in consumption of extreme foods. Black people may have a predisposition for the disease, but it is the way of eating that fosters it.

Sickle cells are caused by an excess of poor-quality yin foods in the diet. To relieve this condition, one should eliminate these foods, and begin following the standard macrobiotic way of eating.

3. Hemophilia

This is a condition in which blood does not clot at its normal rate. Hemophiliacs may bleed excessively from minor injuries such as small cuts, and when they receive even a light blow, large black and blue spots appear under the skin. Normally, when blood flows from any place in the body, it immediately coagulates; but in hemophilia this does not happen. Blood, which is yang, normally forms a resinous type of substance when it comes in contact with oxygen. If this does not occur, however, the blood is in a very yin condition.

Hemophilia is considered to be hereditary, often occuring repeatedly in the same family. Many members of the old imperial families of Europe, like the Hapsburgs and Romanoffs, were afflicted with it. Hemophilia is caused not by heredity but by improper diet. In cases like the Romanoffs and Hapsburgs, it resulted from a rich diet and luxurious lifestyle, both of which produce an excessively yin condition, in which the red blood cells become weak and so do the blood vessels. The red blood cells lose their ability to attract the oxygen needed for coagulation, and the blood vessels do not have the power to fuse or close once they have been ruptured. Foods like animal fats, butter, and eggs accelerate this condition by making the blood more acidic. Hemophilia occurs more in men than in women. This is because women are internally more yang than men, and can therefore absorb more of their opposite without becoming unbalanced.

Medical science considers hemophilia incurable and has no method of treatment. The best advice that doctors can give is to avoid injuries. Although it may take several years, hemophilia can be cured through proper eating. The standard macrobiotic way of eating, with a slight emphasis toward more contractive foods, is the remedy for this disease. Plenty of good physical activity is also recommended.

4. Rh Incompatibility

The blood of many people contains a substance known as the "Rh factor." The name "Rh" came from the Rhesus monkey, which was used in the initial experiments connected with this problem. This factor, called "Rh positive," is found in about 85% of the population. If it is missing, the blood is described as "Rh negative." The Rh factor acts as an agglutinogen, which means that it causes a clumping together of red blood cells. When Rh positive blood is transfused into someone with Rh negative, the body of the recipient produces an anti-Rh agglutinogen, usually within two weeks after the transfusion. Serious difficulties may arise if this person is given a second transfusion. The presence of this anti-agglutinogen results in a hemolytic reaction, or the destruction of red blood cells, which can be fatal.

If the fetus of an Rh negative woman is Rh positive, the anti-Rh factor produced by her body as a defense mechanism may pass through the placenta to the fetus. The baby may then experience a hemolytic reaction in which its red blood cells are destroyed. This is usually fatal.

Since the Rh factor produces agglutination, Rh positive blood is more yang, while Rh negative is more yin. When Rh positive blood is transfused into Rh negative, the anti-Rh factor arises. This means that the more yin blood can tolerate only a small amount of yang. In this case, however, with a second transfusion, the blood of the recipient becomes very yang, triggering the hemolytic reaction. This happens because the red blood cells cannot tolerate this second influx of yang, since like repels like. In order to balance this, the red blood cells suddenly expand and decompose.

The Rh factor of the blood can be changed more easily through proper eating than can the blood type. This is because blood type reflects a person's constitution, whereas the Rh factor represents the condition. Through dietary adjustment, Rh positive blood can become Rh negative and vice versa.

Recently the number of people with Rh positive blood has been increasing. This Rh positive and Rh negative differentiation is caused by present eating patterns. In other words, the modern diet is extreme on both sides. About 48% of the average daily diet in America is comprised of animal foods, including dairy. This necessitates eating large quantities of carbohydrates to make balance. Usually large amounts of simple sugar—either in the form of refined cane sugar, maple sugar, refined flour, and fruits, are used to achieve this. However, if we eat a more balanced or neutral diet, our blood reflects this balance and the Rh factor will be neither strongly positive or negative. If you receive a transfusion under these circumstances, an extreme reaction between plus and minus factors should not arise. In this case the difference between the blood of a mother and her baby will not be great enough to produce an extreme reaction. Persons not eating properly should be very careful about this problem, however.

5. Acidosis and Alkalosis

The acid or alkaline quality of the blood depends upon the concentration of hydrogen (H+) ions and hydroxyl (OH—) ions in our system. These should be balanced. The pH factor, ranging in a scale from pH—1 to pH—12, measures this condition. A pH of less than 7 is acid, while more than 7 is alkaline. Our blood should be slightly alkaline, with a pH between 7.3 and 7.45. If the pH of the blood dips below its normally weak alkaline level, and becomes acidic, the yin condition of acidosis arises. The more yang condition of alkalosis occurs when the pH factor of the blood moves into the high pH range. Of the two, acidosis is more common, since, being yang, humans have a tendency to seek their opposite.

Although many of us continuously eat acidic foods, our blood maintains a weak alkaline condition, as the result of several bodily mechanisms. For example, when we exhale, acids are discharged along with carbon dioxide, and the kidneys continuously filter acids from the blood and discharge them through urination. Also, our blood contains a variety of buffers which serve to neutralize acids. A typical buffer action is illustrated as follows:

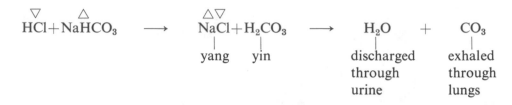

$$\overset{\triangledown}{HCl} + \overset{\triangle}{NaHCO_3} \longrightarrow \overset{\triangle\triangledown}{NaCl} + H_2CO_3 \longrightarrow H_2O + CO_3$$

NaCl: yang | H_2CO_3: yin

H_2O discharged through urine | CO_3 exhaled through lungs

In this reaction, a strong acid (HCl) is replaced by a weak acid (H_2CO_3). This weaker acid is then broken down into water and carbon dioxide, which are then discharged respectively through urination and breathing. Since hydrochloric acid is yin, it attracts yang in the form of sodium bicarbonate ($NaHCO_3$) as it enters the bloodstream. Sodium is the most yang component of this compound. It attracts chlorine, which is the most yin component of the acid. This results in the formation of sodium chloride (NaCl) plus a weak carbonic acid, which, as we have already seen, is easily broken down and discharged. The body uses this buffer response to eliminate the acid formed when we consume simple sugar.

The best way to avoid acidosis or alkalosis is to maintain a neutral or balanced blood condition through proper eating. When correctly applied, the standard macrobiotic way of eating will result in the maintenance of a balanced, slightly alkaline condition.

The Circulatory System

There are seven major divisions of the circulatory system (see Fig. 45.):
1. Circuit through the heart (coronary circuit)
2. Circuit through the upper extremities (shoulders, arms)
3. Circuit through the neck and head
4. Circuit through the thorax (lungs)
5. Circuit through the abdominal area (digestive organs)
6. Circuit though the kidneys (renal circuit)
7. Circuit through the pelvis and lower extremities (legs)

The circulatory system can be compared to a tree. Each of its major circuits fork into numerous smaller branches which in turn divide into millions of peripheral capillaries. Ultimately, the capillaries differentiate into the trillions of cells within the body. The central regions of the circulatory system can be likened to the bough and stem of a tree, while the peripheral regions correspond to the branches and leaves. The body's cells comprise the most peripheral part of the circulatory system, and correspond to the tree's fruit.

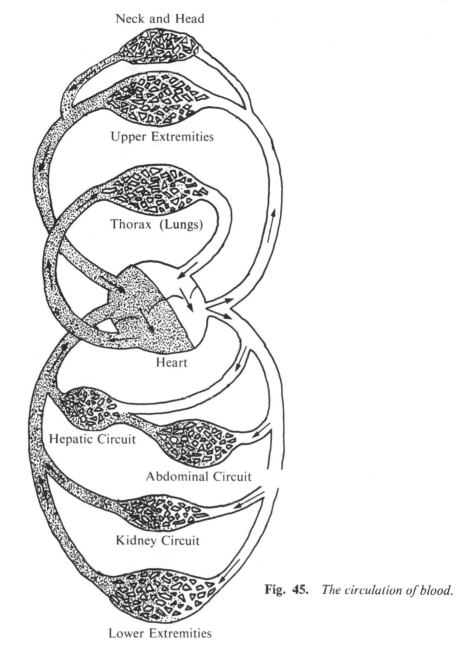

Fig. 45. *The circulation of blood.*

The Macrobiotic Approach to Cardiovascular Diseases

1. Arteriosclerosis (Hardening of the Arteries)

This condition occurs when the insides of the arteries become clogged and lose their normal elasticity. It is caused by the accumulation of cholesterol and fat. In severe cases, the passageway in the arteries becomes progressively narrow and eventually closes. The resulting blockage of blood flow usually causes a heart attack and often death.

As we saw in the chapter, *The Progressive Development of Sickness*, fat and cholesterol deposits result from the repeated consumption of foods such as meat and saturated fat, eggs, dairy products, sugar, refined and processed grain products, and others. This condition used to be rare in persons under the age of 50, but now it is even found among school-age children.

To determine whether you have this condition, put the fingers of both hands together and try to push them back to an angle of 90 degrees. If they cannot go this far, your arteries are hard and inflexible. The dietary approach for the relief of this condition is discussed below.

2. Stroke (Cerebral Hemorrhage or Thrombosis)

A cerebral hemorrhage is caused by the weakening of the blood vessels. When a person with this condition is in a relaxed state there is usually no problem. However, any sudden increase in circulation may cause a weak blood vessel to burst. When this happens in one of the blood vessels in the brain, it is called a "cerebral hemorrhage" or "stroke." The second type of stroke is called "cerebral thrombosis" and results from a clot or blockage in one of the blood vessels in the brain. This condition is generally caused by the same types of foods that produce arteriosclerosis, and often occurs when deposited fat or cholesterol breaks loose from the wall of an artery and lodges in one of the cranial blood vessels.

To relieve these conditions, foods which weaken the blood vessels or which create fat or cholesterol deposits should be avoided. These include saturated fats like those contained in meat, eggs, and dairy prodcuts, as well as sugar and other strong yin foods. Mineral-rich foods like seaweeds and hard leafy vegetables will restore the blood vessels to their normal strength and flexibility, while the standard macrobiotic way of eating will gradually melt the deposits of fat and cholesterol away. A person with these disorders must limit his intake of oil, and should use only unsaturated vegetable oils such as sesame or corn oil. This general approach can also be applied for arteriosclerosis.

3. Abnormal Blood Pressure (Hypertension and Hypotension)

An excessive intake of liquid and other types of yin often causes the heart to become swollen and expanded. In this condition, the organ must work harder in order to maintain the normal circulation of blood, and often *hypertension*, or high blood pressure, results. If a person with this condition continues to take excess yin, the heart may become so swollen and loose that it no longer has sufficient contracting power. As a result, blood pressure often becomes dangerously low, producing what is called *hypotension*.

Hypertension is less serious than hypotension, and can be cured in about one month through proper eating, whereas hypotension is a more advanced symptom and therefore takes a longer time to cure. Since both conditions are the result of over-expansion, within the standard macrobiotic way of eating, we should emphasize more yang factors in our cooking and selection of food.

4. Dilation of an Arterial Wall (Aneurysm)

This condition arises when the wall of an artery expands and creates a small sac which fills with blood. This occurs when an artery has become weak from the intake of yin, and happens most often in the aorta, since the blood pressure there is very high and yin factors are readily attracted to this region. This condition can be overcome through the standard macrobiotic way of eating, with a little more salt and oil than usual in cooking. These factors have the effect of making the arteries more elastic.

5. Broken Capillaries

When the blood vessels become swollen and enlarged from the overconsumption of yin, they start to break down. The functions between branches are particularly susceptible. Nosebleeding is a good example of this. It occurs when the blood becomes too thin and when its volume becomes excessive. The direct cause is often the overintake of fruit juice, soda, water, and other liquids. Nosebleeding can be quickly relieved by making the blood thicker and the capillaries more contracted. To do this, moisten a piece of tissue or paper napkin with saliva and dip it in salt or *dentie*. Insert this in your nostril for several minutes. Also, to quickly thicken the blood, eat a small amount of *gomasio* or a piece of *umeboshi* plum every 10 minutes for about one-half hour.

6. Artherosclerosis

This is a type of arteriosclerosis in which deposits of fat develop within and around the heart. These deposits start in the more peripheral regions of the circulatory system and gradually move inward. The cause of this condition is the same as that for arteriosclerosis—in other words, foods which contribute to the development of fat and cholesterol. We should therefore approach it in the same way as arteriosclerosis.

Twenty-five years ago, heart disease affected about one out of eight people. This rate has increased tremendously, so that now, at least two out of every five people will eventually develop it. One out of every three men and one out of every six women in the Unites States can be expected to die of heart disease or stroke before the age of 60. It is now known that saturated fats and cholesterol are largely responsible for these disorders, and many medical associations have advised the avoidance of fat as well as an overall reduction of cholesterol-rich foods like meat and eggs. However, these recommendations usually overlook the other types of foods which contribute to these problems, such as sugar, fruits, and dairy foods.

The Lymphatic System

The blood and lymphatic systems are closely related. The bloodstream is generally more yang and its main function is to transport red blood cells. The lymph stream, carrying a clearer liquid, is more yin, and deals primarily with the white blood cells. Both comprise the circulatory system as a whole, and circulate in opposite yet complementary directions. Blood circulation begins in the heart, radiates outward to the more peripheral regions, and then returns. Conversely, the flow of lymph begins in the peripheral body tissues, and then enters the central bloodstream.

Unlike the bloodstream the lymphatic system has no central organ to pump the lymph fluid. The flow of lymph is maintained by several factors, such as the activity and contraction of the muscles. Another factor is the action of the lungs and diaphragm during breathing, which has the effect of "sucking" lymph from the smaller vessels into the larger vessels, while the tendency of yin liquid to rise causes the lymph to flow from the lower to the upper parts of the body. Also, the function of the intestines, including the movements of the villi and the contractions of the intestine as a whole, contribute to the flow of lymph. Since the villi are continuously taking in digested food particles, these are continuously flowing into both the blood and lymph streams, along with newly created red and white blood cells.

The lymphatic system consists of lymph capillaries, vessels, ducts, and nodes, as well as such organs as the tonsils and spleen. The lymph nodes are found at intervals throughout the lymphatic system, and are arranged in 32 paired groups, correlating to the 32 teeth and spinal vertebrae. The lymphatic system also contains another major organ which is located above the heart. Known as the thymus, this organ reaches its largest size at the age of two, and then gradually declines until it disappears entirely. The thymus produces white blood cells along with certain types of antibodies.

The spleen is the major organ of the lymphatic system. Located opposite the liver on the left side of the body, it has the following functions:
1. Filtration and cleansing of lymph and body fluid. The spleen filters substances like bacteria and worn-out red blood cells from these fluids.
2. Formation of white blood cells, especially lymphocytes.
3. Storage of blood and minerals, particularly iron.
4. Productin of antibodies (immunization factors). These are very important in the body's natural resistance to bacteria.
5. Bile production.

The liver and spleen are complementary. The liver is yang in comparison, and functions in coordination with the bloodstream, while the spleen, which is more yin, serves as the major focus of the lymphatic system. The major function of the lymphatic system is to keep the body clean through the removal of toxic excess.

The Macrobiotic Approach to Diseases of the Lymphatic System

1. Hodgkin's Disease and Lymphosarcoma

These diseases are similar to leukemia. In Hodgkin's disease, the lymph nodes and spleen become inflamed, while in lymphosarcoma, a malignant tumor develops within the lymphoid tissue, and the lymphatic organs become swollen. As with leukemia, both diseases involve an increase in the number of white blood cells. The cause of both is similar to the cause of leukemia, namely, an excessive intake of yin foods, along with a corresponding deficiency in the factors necessary for the production of red blood cells. The way of controlling both conditions is similar to that for leukemia and other types of yin cancer, and is outlined in the chapter, *The Progressive Development of Sickness.*

2. Tonsillitis

This illness occurs when the lymphatic system localizes various types of toxic excess in the tonsils. Suppose, for example, someone eats a large quantity of ice cream or other extreme food. Immediately the lymphatic system begins to localize this excess for discharging. Additional white blood cells are created in the tonsils to neutralize any harmful bacteria that may form, while minerals start to gather in this region as a buffer for the discharge of acids. In the meantime, the tonsils may become inflamed and the body temperature may rise. If, at this time, the person has the tonsils removed, the fever and inflammation may disappear, but the toxic bodily fluids will continue to circulate throughout the system, and the remaining lymphatic organs will have to work much harder to perform the discharge function of the tonsils. The net result is a reduction in the ability of the lymphatic system to efficiently rid the body of toxic excess. This will not necessarily cause serious problems, provided the person eats properly. However, if the person continues to eat poorly, he will begin to experience a lack of vitality. A person in this condition is more susceptible to illness, and has less self-healing ability than someone who has not had his tonsils removed. The relationship between operations such as tonsilectomies and the development of illnesses such as cancer and multiple sclerosis is discussed elsewhere in this book.

3. General Lymphatic Troubles

These can be summarized into two types:
1. Expansion or inflammation of the lymphatic nodes and organs. In extreme cases, this leads to a rupture of the lymphatic vessels. These problems result when the lymph fluid contains too much fatty acid.
2. Hardening of the nodes, organs, ducts, and capillaries.

To relieve these problems, observe the standard macrobiotic way of eating. A hot ginger compress can be applied over the afflicted area to activate circulation and can be followed by a taro potato plaster. These applications will help to reduce the accompanying fever and melt fat and hardness around the lymph vessels. A *tofu* plaster is also helpful in reducing fever and inflammation. If the problem is chronic, external applications should be used repeatedly until the condition improves, and the patient should eat very well during this time. An operation to correct the condition is unnecessary.

Appendix

Blood Type

It is important to know your blood type, especially in emergencies which require a blood transfusion. There are four major types: O, A, B, and AB. Certain types can be mixed, while others cause "agglutination," which is a clumping together of the blood cells. If you receive the wrong type of blood, death can result. Fig. 46 indicates which types of blood can be combined. The horizontal column indicates the recipient, while the vertical column indicates the donor.

Since, in most cases, people with Type O blood can give to people with any other type, they are classified as universal donors. People with Type AB are the opposite in this respect: they can give only to others of the same type of blood. However, they can receive blood from people with any of the other types. Fig. 47 shows the frequency with which the blood types occur, along with their arrangement from most yang to most yin.

Donor Type:	Recipient Type:	O	A	B	AB
O		yes	yes	yes	yes
A		no	yes	no	yes
B		no	no	yes	yes
AB		no	no	no	yes

Fig. 46.

	Blood Type	White People	Asian-African
Most Yang	O	43%	Same
	B	13%	More
	AB	4%	Same
Most Yin	A	40%	Less

Fig. 47.

Since Type O is the most yang, it can be given to many people. It has been said that people with this type of blood become either beggars or generals, meaning that they have the potential to be either very lazy or very great. A person with Type B is yang, but less so than someone with Type O. Type B individuals tend to be better at speaking than writing, and usually have cheerful, outgoing personalities. Type A individuals are the most yin, and usually have a more inward or gentle personality, and are usually better at work involving details such as accounting and writing. A person with Type AB blood is in between Types A and B, and has characteristics of both.

Blood Pressure

The amount of pressure the blood exerts against the walls of the vessels is described as "blood pressure." Blood pressure fluctuates throughout the body. It is highest in the aorta, and becomes progressively lower in the arteries, capillaries, and veins. There are different types of blood pressure. The general term "blood pressure" refers to the pressure in the major arteries, while venous pressure refers to that in the veins, and capillary pressure to that in the capillaries.

Blood pressure is generally expressed in terms of a fraction such as 120/80, which reads "one-twenty over eighty." The first number records the pressure of the blood during the yang or contracting phase of the heart, and is called the *systolic* pressure. The second number is called the *diastolic* pressure, and records the pressure during the heart's yin, expanded phase. Both figures indicate the level in millimeters reached by a column of mercury which is contained within the measuring instrument. When we take the average of the systolic and diastolic pressures, we obtain what is called the "mean blood pressure." For example, to determine the mean blood pressure in the above example, we would add 120 and 80, and divide the sum by 2. Thus, the mean blood pressure in this case would be 100.

Fig. 48 shows the average blood pressure among young people in the United States for the different regions of the circulatory system.

Blood pressure tends to increase with age. Fig. 49 shows the average variations in systolic pressure according to age.

Persons who consume little or no animal food have blood pressures which are about 10 mm lower than average. This was confirmed several years ago by Dr. Edward Kass, Dr. Frank Sacks, and others at the Harvard University School of Medicine in a study of several hundred macrobiotic people living in the Boston area. The results of this study were published in the *American Journal of Epidemiology* (Vol. 100, No. 5) under the title "Blood Pressure in Vegetarians."*

On the average, the blood pressure of men is between 8 and 10 mm higher than that of women. This indicates that men are more easily excitable than women. When women reach menopause, however, their blood pressure rises to about the same level as men. From this age on, the blood pressure of men and women tend to be equal, with the levels for women tending to be slightly higher.

Arterial	
systolic	110–120
diastolic	65–80
Capillaries	20–30
Veins (those near the heart)	0–20

Fig. 48.

Age	mm
Birth	40
12 months	80
12 years	100
15 ,,	110
20 ,,	120
40 ,,	125
65 ,,	134
Over 65	Increases rapidly

Fig. 49.

* In a later study, this same research team investigated the relationship between diet and blood fat and cholesterol levels. The subjects for this study were a group of people in the Boston area who were following the standard macrobiotic way of eating. The results of this study, published in the *New England Journal of Medicine*, (May 29, 1975), under the title "Plasma Lipids and Lipoproteins in Vegetarians and Controls," demonstrated that these individuals had lower than average blood fat and cholesterol levels, and that the consumption of dairy products and eggs contributed to an increase in these levels.

CHAPTER SEVEN

The Endocrine System

In addition to the highly charged bloodstream and lymphatic system, our body contains other fluids which are also receiving a constant charge of energy from heaven and earth as well as from the meridians. These highly charged liquids can function in either of two ways: (1) to influence the functioning of the organs, in which case they are known as hormones, or (2) to aid in the decomposition of food, in which case they are known as digestive liquids. We can understand how the highly charged digestive liquid decomposes nutrients by considering the model of a water molecule.

A water molecule is composed of one oxygen atom, which is yin, and two hydrogen atoms, which are yang. (See Fig. 50.) However, one of the hydrogen atoms is positively charged, while the other is negative. When a particular substance is placed in water, its more yang components are attracted to water's yin pole, while its more yin components gravitate towards their opposite pole. This process results in the decomposition of the substance, and thus water is often referred to as the "universal solvent."

Another group of these highly charged liquids are known as hormones. The major endocrine glands are located principally along the spiritual channel, with the exception of the adrenal glands, which differentiate off to either side.

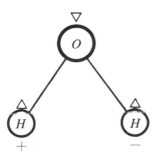

Fig. 50. *In a molecule of water, one atom of oxygen ($\triangledown$) is balanced by two hydrogen atoms ($\triangle$); one of which carries a positive charge, and the other of which carries a negative charge.*

The General Pattern of the Endocrine System

Heaven's downward force enters the body through the spiral on the top of the head. As it passes downward, it charges and activates the midbrain, and also is responsible for the embryonic formation of the uvula. On the other hand, earth's expanding force passes upward through the body, and in the head region its action is responsible for the formation of the tongue. (See Fig. 51.)

Saliva is produced in this region through the interaction of these two forces, serving principally as a highly charged digestive liquid. In ancient spiritual practices, saliva was referred to as "the dew of heaven and earth," and it was often collected in the mouth and then swallowed in order to vitalize the entire body. This highly-charged fluid is naturally generated through proper chewing.

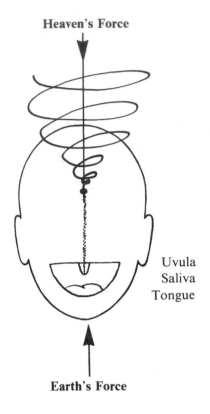

Heaven's Force

Uvula
Saliva
Tongue

Earth's Force

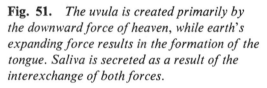

Fig. 51. *The uvula is created primarily by the downward force of heaven, while earth's expanding force results in the formation of the tongue. Saliva is secreted as a result of the interexchange of both forces.*

During the process of biological evolution, we passed through the stage of four-legged mammals. In this form, heaven's force enters through the tail and passes along the spine toward the midbrain. At the same time, it enters through the back of the head, creating another uvula deep within the brain. This "uvula" is known as the *pituitary gland*, and it secretes highly-charged liquid known as *pituitary hormones*. (See Fig. 52.)

The head and the torso have a complementary-antagonistic relationship. What occurs in a compacted form in the head also occurs in the torso in a more expanded form. In the case of the endocrine system, the single pituitary gland located in the compacted head differentiates into multiple endocrine glands in the expanded torso. These differentiations are as follows (see Fig. 53.):

1. *Throat*—The thyroid gland which is more yin; the parathyroid glands which are more yang.
2. *Above Both Kidneys*—The adrenal glands secrete both yin and yang hormones.
3. *Pancreas*—The pancreas also secretes both yin and yang hormones.
4. *Duodenum*—The duodenum mucosa secretes a variety of hormones.
5. *Gonads*—The sexual hormones are of a more yin variety and a more yang variety.
6. *The Placenta*—This arises during pregnancy.

Since these glands are complementary-antagonistic differentiations of the pituitary, they are all influenced by its secretions. For example, suppose you walk past a bakery and notice a cake in the window. The visual image of the cake stimulates the pituitary, which in turn stimulates the thyroid and parathyroid, the secretion of saliva and stomach juices, and the duodenum mucosa which in turn causes the secretion of digestive liquid. These digestive and hormone liquids are already secreted before the cake is eaten.

Another example is when a man catches sight of a beautiful woman. This visual stimulation goes to the midbrain, which in turn activates the pituitary gland. The secretions of the pituitary in turn influence the adrenal glands and the gonads. The result is that the man feels sexually attracted to the woman.

Heaven's force also creates and charges the male sexual organs. In this sense, we can consider the penis as a second uvula. The secretions of the male sexual organs are highly charged with electromagnetic energy, or in other words, very "alive." This is why sperm are capable of self-motion.

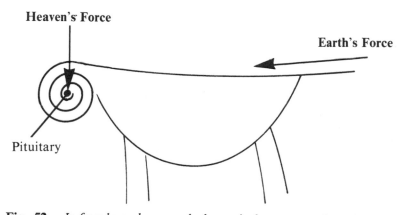

Fig. 52. *In four-legged mammals, heaven's force enters through the tail, especially when it is raised, and the top of the head, where it creates the pituitary gland.*

The Physiology of the Endocrine System

1. Pituitary Gland (Hypophysis Cerebri)

The pituitary gland is located at the base of the brain and consists of an *anterior*, or front, lobe, and a *posterior*, or back, lobe. The anterior lobe secretes the following more yin hormones: (1) *growth hormone*, which regulates growth; (2) *thyrotropic hormone*, which regulates the development and functioning of the thyroid gland; (3) *gonadotropic hormones* which regulate the sex organs; (4) *lactogenic hormone* (prolactin), which initiates the secretion of milk by the mammary glands; and (5) *adrenocorticotropic hormone*, which is essential for the development and activity of the adrenal cortex.

The following more yang hormones are secreted by the posterior lobe: (1) *vaso-pressin* (pitressin or ADH) which causes the blood vessels to contract and inhibits urination, and (2) *oxygocin* which causes the uterus to contract.

These are the major known hormones which are secreted by the pituitary gland. There are probably others which have not as yet been identified.

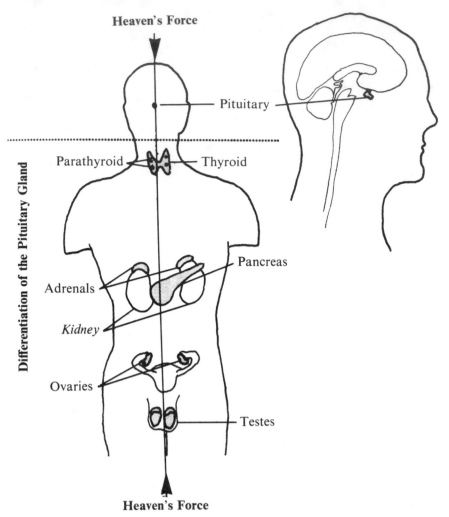

Fig. 53. *In the human body, the single pituitary gland differentiates below the neck into the thyroid and parathyroid glands, the adrenal glands, the pancreatic alpha and beta cells, the duodenum mucosa, the gonads, and during pregnancy, into the placenta.*

2. Thyroid and Parathyroid Glands

These glands are located in the area of the throat *chakra*. The more yang parathyroid glands (usually four in number) lie within the thyroid gland, which is larger and more expanded. The thyroid and parathyroid glands have a complementary and antagonistic relationship.

The thyroid secretes the hormone *thyroxin* which regulate the body's basal metabolism, or the rate of cellular oxydation. The parathyroid glands secrete *parathormone* which controls the metabolism of minerals such as calcium and phosphorous.

3. Adrenal Glands

The adrenal glands are located on top of both kidneys, and are separated into a more peripheral region known as the *cortex*, and a more central region known as the *medulla*. More yin hormones are secreted by the cortex, while the medulla secretes hormones which are more yang.

The structure of the cortex is more differentiated than that of the medulla. The cortex secretes a variety of hormones most notably those known as *steroids*. These regulate the metabolism of ingested proteins, fats, and carbohydrates, as well as the body's water and salt balance. Aside from regulating the metabolism of nutrients, this group of hormones also stimulate the functioning of the parasympathetic branch of the autonomic nerve.

The medulla secretes two hormones: *adrenalin*, or ephinephrine, and *noradrenalin*, or norephinephrine, which influence various bodily functions in a manner similar to that brought about by stimulation of the orthosympathetic nerve.

The adrenal glands, which are centrally located within the body, have a very important role within the endocrine system. The greatest complementarity within the endocrine system exists between the pituitary and the adrenal glands. All of the other endocrine glands can be considered as branches of these.

4. Pancreas

The pancreas has the double function of secreting both digestive juices and hormones. These hormones are secreted in the region of the pancreas known as the *islets of Langerhans*. Within the islets, two main types of cells can be distinguished: small *beta* cells which secrete a more yang hormone known as *insulin*, and larger *alpha* cells which secrete a more yin hormone known as *glucagon*, or anti-insulin. Both hormones affect the metabolism of carbohydrates. Insulin lowers the blood sugar level, while glucagon causes it to rise, by stimulating the liver to release glucose.

5. Duodenum

The surface of the duodenum secretes several hormones which influence the functioning of the pancreas, liver, gall bladder, and stomach. Among these are:
1. *Secretin*, which brings about the secretion of pancreatic juice and increases the flow of bile in the liver;
2. *Pancreozymin*, which also stimulates the secretion of pancreatic juice;
3. *Cholecystokinin*, which causes the gall bladder to contract and thereby discharge bile;
4. *Enterogasterone*, which limits the activity of the stomach, including the secretion of stomach acid.

The duodenum is a more compacted part of the digestive system, and the hormones that it secretes are generally yang, although they differ in degree; and they have an antagonistic relationship to the more expanded parts of the body such as the stomach wall. Since it is longer and wider, the small intestine secretes intestinal juice which is more yin.

6. Gonads

These are male of female, and their hormones differ accordingly. The female hormones are created principally in the ovaries, while the testes produce the male hormones.

A. The Ovaries.   The ovarian follicle, a spirallically-formed mass of cells in which the ovum develops, secretes a group of hormones known as *estrogens*. Also called the "female" hormones, estrogens play an essential role in the development of female characteristics and in the maintenance of sexual libido. Estrogens are widely known as a result of their use in birth control pills, and are more yin.

Progesterone is secreted by the corpus luteum, which is the mass of cells that develop within a ruptured follicle following ovulation. Under the influence of progesterone, the uterus prepares to receive the fertilized ovum. If implantation occurs, progesterone induces the formation of the placenta. Progesterone is the most yang of the female hormones.

B. The Testis.   Male hormones are known as *androgens*, the most important of which is *testosterone*. This hormone regulates the development of male characteristics which occur at puberty such as the growth of facial hair and the deepening of the voice. Testosterone is a yang hormone.

7. Placenta

During pregnancy, the placenta secretes the following hormones: (1) *chorionic gonadotrophin*, (2) estrogens, and (3) progesterone. Chorionic gonadotrophin forms the basis of various pregnancy tests, since it appears in the blood and urine of women within two weeks after fertilization. This hormone stimulates the formation of the placenta and is produced only after the fertilized ovum is implanted. During pregnancy, the placenta also assumes the production of both estrogens and progesterone.

A Summary of the Endocrine System

The principal endocrine glands are summarized in the following chart:

HEAD
Pituitary Gland

▽

Anterior Lobe
growth hormone
thyrotropic
gonadotropic
lactogenic
adrenocorticotropic

△

Posterior Lobe
vasopressin (ADH)
oxytocin

BODY

▽	△
Thyroid	**Parathyroid**
thyroxin	parathormone
Adrenal Cortex	**Adrenal Medulla**
steroids	adrenalin
Pancreatic Alpha Cells	**Pancreatic Beta Cells**
glucagon	insulin
Gastric and Intestinal Juice	**Duodenal Hormones**
Ovaries	**Testis**
estrogen ▽	androgen
progesterone △	

The single pituitary gland differentiates in the lower body into the following eight major functions: (1) thyroid, (2) parathyroid, (3) adrenal cortex and (4) medulla, (5) pancreatic alpha and (6) beta cells, (7) gonads, and (8) duodenal mucosa. In general, the more yang hormones of the endocrine system show a relation to the functioning of the sympathetic nerve, while the more yin hormones are related to the parasympathetic nerve.

The central function of the hormone system is to regulate and control the use of food, including the digestion of solid food, the intake and use of oxygen, and the metabolism and balance of carbohydrates, fats, proteins, minerals, and water. These functions, which result in the growth of the body, the maintenance of vitality, and the ability to reproduce, are summarized in the following chart:

Pituitary Gland
GROWTH

1. **Thyroid**	2. **Parathyroid**
O_2 metabolism	mineral metabolism
	3. **Adrenals**
VITALITY	CH, fat, protein metabolism; salt and water balance
5. **Duodenum**	4. **Pancreas**
digestion	sugar metabolism

REPRODUCTION

Male testis	**Female ovaries**

Diseases of the Endocrine System

In general, there are two basic types of endocrine disfunctions: (1) hyposecretion, in which not enough of a particular hormone is secreted, and (2) hypersecretion, in which too much is secreted. Either of these can result in an unbalanced condition, in the following manner:

1. *Hyposecretion of a yin hormone produces an overly yang condition.*
2. *Hyposecretion of a yang hormone produces an overly yin condition.*
3. *Hypersecretion of a yin hormone produces an overly yin condition.*
4. *Hypersecretion of a yang hormone produces an overly yang condition.*

Let us now consider specific disfunction in each of the major endocrine glands.

1. Pituitary

Hyposecretion of an expansive hormone such as growth hormone will result in *dwarfism*, if it begins from an early age, or, if it begins at a later age, in *pituitary cachexia;* both situations are overly-yang conditions. Hyposecretion of an opposite type of hormone such as vasopressin (ADH) creates a condition known as *diabetes insipidis*, which is an excessive loss of body fluids due to a great increase in the frequency of urination.

Hypersecretion of an expansive hormone such as growth hormone, if from an early age, creates *giantism*, while if it begins at a later age, a condition known as *acromegaly*. Hypersecretion of an opposite type of hormone such as ADH results in a condition in which urination is difficult.

2. Thyroid

Hyposecretion of thyroxin can result in: (1) *simple goiter*, which is an enlargement of the thyroid gland resulting primarily from a lack of iodine in the diet, and (2) *mydexedema*, or *Gull's disease* in an adult, and *cretinism* during childhood. Both mydexedema and cretinism have common symptoms such as physical and mental retardation, abnormal metabolism, low body temperature, slow heartbeat, and thickened skin. With mydexedema, the nose becomes swollen and a loss of hair occurs.

These conditions can result from either the overconsumption of yin foods or the overconsumption of yang foods.

Hypersecretion of thyroxin can produce *exophthalmic goiter (Graves' disease)* or *toxic goiter*. Exophthalmic goiter is characterized by a swollen throat, an increase in the metabolic rate, a rapid heartbeat, muscular weakness, shortness of breath, and various nervous disturbances, irritability, tremors, and protruding eyeballs. Toxic goiter results from a tumor in the thyroid and the symptoms are generally the same as for exophthalmic goiter, with the exception of protruding eyeballs.

3. Parathyroid

Hyposecretion of parathormone results in a decrease in the concentration of calcium in the blood. This condition is known as *tetany* and results in cramps and muscle spasms. Hypersecretion of parathormone causes calcium to be drawn from the bones and discharged into the blood. This condition, known as *osteitis fibrosa*, may lead to extensive changes in the bone structure, skeletal deformities, and the deposit of calcium in the kidneys.

4. Adrenals

Sicknesses of the medulla are not very common. Adrenal disorders arise more frequently in the cortex. Hyposecretion of the cortex causes *Addison's disease*, which is marked by a degeneration of the cortex region, causing fatigue, low blood pressure, reduced basal metabolism, muscular debility, abnormal pigmentation of the skin, etc. This sickness results from the overconsumption of animal products and salt, as well as from overeating.

Hypersecretion of the cortex which occurs during pregnancy or childhood can result in *sexual precocity*, or the failure of the sexual organs to develop. If this condition occurs later in life, it can result in the tendency to reverse sexes.

5. Pancreas

Hyposecretion of insulin results in *diabetes mellitus*, while hypersecretion causes *hyperinsulinism*. Both of these will be discussed extensively at the end of this chapter.

6. Testis and Ovaries

Hyposecretion of the testis results in a decrease in sexual appetite. In the ovaries, hyposecretion of estrogen can cause the uterus to atrophy and the sexual libido to decline. Hyposecretion of progesterone results in menstrual disorders and the tendency toward miscarriage.

Hypersecretion of the testis or ovaries can result in an abnormal desire for sex.

Endocrine disorders are not difficult to diagnose. For example, various troubles in the upper region of the body such as bulging eyes, ear problems, mental disorders, and others are related to dysfunction of the pituitary and/or the thyroid. Disorders in the lower region of the body such as poor digestion, sexual troubles, and others are all related to problems of the adrenals or lower endocrine glands. All sicknesses are related to dysfunction of the endocrine system. Even problems like acne or pimples indicate that an excess of yin hormones are being released into the blood.

The Macrobiotic Approach to Endocrine Diseases

1. Dietary Approach

The principles for approaching endocrine disorders are as follows: (1) In cases where not enough of a particular yin hormone is secreted, or if an excess of a yang hormone is secreted, the patient should eat a slightly more yin diet. (2) When the body is not producing enough of a particular yang hormone, or if too much of a yin hormone is produced, the patient should eat a slightly more yang diet. Of course, the standard macrobiotic way of eating should form the basis upon which these minor adjustments can be made. For example, for a more yin condition the proportion of sesame seeds to salt in *gomasio* should be about 10 to 1 or 8 to 1; for a more yang condition, about 12 or 15 to 1. A person with a yin disorder should have a slightly stronger tasting *miso* soup, while a lighter *miso* soup should be served to someone with the opposite condition. Among vegetables, green leafy vegetables are good for someone who is overly-yang, while root vegetables should be emphasized by someone with a more yin condition.

As a practical illustration, suppose a woman is suffering from a condition in which not enough estrogen is produced. To relieve this condition, animal products should be avoided, cooking should be light, green leafy vegetables should be emphasized, and an occasional small volume of fruit may be eaten. An opposite type of condition results when too much estrogen is secreted, or when a woman has taken birth control pills. In this case, a slightly more yang diet will bring relief.

If a man lacks sexual vitality, or develops female characteristics, this results primarily from the over-intake of sugar and dairy products. In this case, root vegetables should be emphasized, salad should be avoided, a little more *miso*, *tamari*, and salt can be used, and fish or other animal products may occasionally be eaten.

2. External Applications

External applications, particularly ginger compresses, can be used to accelerate the activity of the pancreas, adrenals, thyroid, or parathyroids. For example, a ginger compress can be applied once a day to the area of the pancreas to help treat diabetes. This should be continued for two to four weeks so as to activate the blood circulation and *ki* flow.

3. Meridian Treatments

Since the endocrine glands receive a constant charge of electromagnetic energy from the environment, we can accelerate their functioning by stimulating the meridians. This can be accomplished through *shiatsu* massage, moxa, or with needles. Although it is not absolutely necessary to supplement the dietary treatment of endocrine disorders with these techniques or with external applications, they will serve to accelerate the cure. To locate the specific points indicated below by number, please refer to an acupuncture chart or text that uses the standard numbering system.

A. Pituitary.   To approach problems occurring in this gland, use the following points on the governing vessel meridian: (1) GV20 (also known as the "hundred meeting" point), (2) GV15, (3) GV16, and (4) GV12, which can also be used in the treatment of multiple sclerosis. The point on the front of the head corresponding to the "third eye" can also be used.

B. Thyroid and Parathyroid.   Any of the major points on the lung meridian can be used to treat thyroid or parathyroid troubles. Like the lungs, these glands are located in the upper region of the body, and they are also involved in the metabolism of oxygen. These glands are also related to the tongue, which is in turn related to the stomach. Therefore, any of the major points on the stomach meridian can also be used.

C.   Adrenals.   The adrenals can be approached by using either the kidney or bladder meridian. A particularly effective way to activate the adrenals is to use *shiatsu* (finger pressure) massage on the bladder meridian running along either side of the spine.

D.   Duodenum.   The duodenum is connected to the stomach, pancreas, gall bladder, and liver. The beginning or end points of these meridians which are located on the toes are very effective for treatment. For the liver or spleen meridian, use the first toe; for the stomach meridian, use the second or third toe; and for the gall bladder meridian, use the fourth toe.

E.   Pancreas.   Pancreatic troubles can be approached through the spleen meridian, as well as its complementary-antagonistic partner, the stomach. The more peripheral regions of these meridians are the most effective in this case, particularly the first, second, or third toes as well as the area of the meridian below the knee.

F.   Gonads.   To treat disorders in these organs, use either the kidney or bladder meridian.

Diabetes Mellitus

This condition, which affects millions of people, is caused by the failure of the islets of Langerhans to produce enough insulin. Hyposecretion of insulin, a yang hormone, results in an overly-yin blood condition in which the level of sugar in the blood rises markedly. This condition is known as hyperglycemia. In normal circumstances, the sugar content of the blood is about 100 mg (70 mg–120 mg) per 100 cc. Fatigue and tiredness begin if this level rises to over 130 mg, and if it increases to 180 mg, what is known as the *renal threshold* is reached. At this point, sugar begins to appear in the urine (glycosuria) and the discharge of urine increases (polyuria). The loss of water through excessive urination causes the patient to become thirsty, while the accompanying loss of glucose and minerals produces hunger.

   Since the metabolism of sugar is disturbed in diabetes, the oxidation of fats, which depends on the oxidation of glucose, does not proceed smoothly. Partially oxidized fats give rise to what are known as *ketone bodies*, and *acetone* (C_3H_6O) appears in the urine, often giving rise to an acetone smell in the breath. Other types of acidic ketone bodies are also formed in large quantities, and this condition necessitates the maintenance of a constant buffer action which depletes the body's mineral reserves. This situation leads to the development of acidosis, and disrupts the metabolism of carbon dioxide. Since carbon dioxide cannot be discharged smoothly, it becomes like a toxin in the body, resulting in possible convulsions, coma, and death.

   A high blood sugar level also has the effect of weakening the peripheral parts of the body, especially the skin. Wounds heal slowly, skin ulcers often develop, the skin loses its natural flexibility and begins to harden, and the circulation becomes poor in the hands and feet. Since diabetes results in a depletion of minerals, the structure of the teeth becomes weak. Also, various eye disorders such as glaucoma are often associated with diabetes.

In the past, diabetes was considered as a disease of old age, since it was more common in persons over 60, arising in many cases after a person achieved material success and could afford gourmet-style food. Presently, however, diabetes arises at any age, and many young people have begun to develop it.

The present medical treatment of diabetes is to inject insulin, but this does not cure the disease. Since the intake of carbohydrates affects the utilization of insulin, the dosage must be adapted to the patient's diet and activity. In many cases, diabetics are placed on a low-carbohydrate and high fat and protein diet. An overdose of insulin may result in insulin shock, convulsions, coma, and in some cases, death, while not enough will leave the patient with diabetic symptoms. It is very dfficult to maintain the correct dosage of insulin, and patients must be checked often and have their dosage adjusted. Recently, it has been found that insulin combined with protamine and zinc is absorbed more slowly, thus requiring less frequent injections, and several oral medicines, most notably *orinase*, have been found somewhat effective in controlling the blood sugar level.

1. The Cause of Diabetes

The cause of diabetes is not known medically. However, with the unifying principle of yin and yang, the solution to this problem is quite easy. Insulin is secreted in the pancreas by the islets of Langerhans. These masses of cells are scattered throughout the pancreas, and vary in number from 200,000 to 1,800,000. They are most numerous in the tail portion of the pancreas.

The more yang beta cells within the islets secrete insulin, while larger and more yin alpha cells secrete glucagon. In diabetes, the beta cells become expanded, and lose their ability to secrete insulin. This is caused by an overly yin blood condition which results from the over-consumption of sugar, fruit, dairy, chemicals, and other similar foods, as well as by the overconsumption of animal products which create an acidic condition.

2. The Macrobiotic Approach to Diabetes

A. Dietary Approach.   The macrobiotic approach to diabetes aims at restoring the capacity of the beta cells to produce insulin by restoring them to a more normal condition. This is accomplished by making the patient's diet slightly more yang as well as through physical activity. The patient's diet should not be too yang, however, since this will cause an attraction to the opposite types of foods, which caused the diabetes to develop in the first place.

A diabetic patient should avoid all of the foods listed as being overly yin or overly yang in the chapter, *The Progressive Development of Sickness*, and should stay within the range of foods included in the standard macrobiotic way of eating. Whole cereal grains should comprise at least 50%, and up to 60%, of the patient's diet. More yang grains such as short grain rice, millet, and buckwheat are particularly advisable. Millet contains plenty of B-vitamins, which serve as a catalyst in the formation of hormones such as insulin, and the patient should often cook a 50-50 or 80-20 rice-millet combination. Grains should be cooked with a small amount of sea salt.

Gomasio should be a little more yang, perhaps 8 to 1 or 10 to 1, while the patient should have only one cup or small bowl of soup per day. *Miso* or *tamari* soup should have a slightly salty taste, but not too salty. Soup should comprise about 5% of the daily diet.

Vegetables should comprise between 20% and 25% of the daily intake. These should primarily be sautéed in oil and seasoned with a little more salt than usual. If the patient becomes thirsty, rather than reducing the amount of salt, increase the amount of oil. More yang oils, such as sesame or corn oil, should be used primarily. Among vegetables, root vegetables like carrots, burdock, and others are best, while round vegetables which grow above the surface of the ground, like onions and cabbage, should also be used. Greens should be selected according to shape, with preference given to small-leafed greens which are hard and have a more complex leaf structure. Kale, *daikon* greens, carrot greens, watercress, parsley, and others fall into this category.

Beans should comprise 10%–15% of the diet, with preference given to smaller beans such as *azukis* and lentils. Chickpeas are too yin for a diabetic patient. Only about 3%–4% seaweed should be eaten, but this should be taken regularly in order to provide a continual supply of minerals.

A diabetic patient should avoid fruit, even if it is cooked. A sweet taste is provided by the complex polysaccharide glucose found in grains, as well as in vegetables like fall and winter squash, pumpkin and carrots. An occasional dessert made of *azuki* beans sweetened with rice honey or barley malt may also be eaten for sweetness.

A diabetic patient should eat a special dish made from 50% hard squash, 30% *azuki* beans, and 20% *kombu* seaweed. These should be cooked together and seasoned with sea salt. Several drops of sesame oil can be added while the dish is being cooked. This combination tastes very sweet, and the patient should eat a portion about the size of a baseball at every meal.

The patient may also have salty pickles, but these should be traditionally prepared and aged for a minimum of three months. Several-day-old pickles are too yin. In general, a person with diabetes should limit his intake of fluid, including the recommended beverages. Roasted grain teas such as those made from barley or rice are especially recommended. A diabetic patient should never eat raw oil, as in salad dressing.

B. Eating Habits. A diabetic patient should chew very thoroughly, preferably between 100 and 200 times per mouthful, and must be careful to avoid overeating and overdrinking. It is better for a diabetic patient to eat small quantities four or five times a day than to eat a single large meal. A person with this condition should also not eat for several hours before going to bed.

C. Lifestyle. Plenty of physical activity is important for a diabetic patient, but this activity should not be overly strenuous. Long hot baths or showers, as well as bathing too frequently, will cause the patient to lose minerals and become very weak. A quick hot bath or shower or a sponge bath is preferable if not taken too often. If a patient feels faint after taking a bath, a cup of *tamari-bancha* tea or a pinch of *gomasio* will help to restore strength.

A diabetic patient should try to get up early every morning. Sleeping late will cause the patient's condition to remain weak.

D. External Applications. Hot ginger compresses as well as the meridian treatments which are described in this chapter are helpful in accelerating the patient's recovery.

E. Medication. A diabetic should continue his normal dosage of insulin during the first two weeks of beginning to eat macrobiotically. As the condition of the pancreas improves, its natural ability to secrete insulin will gradually return, during which period the patient can gradually reduce the dosage of insulin. The patient should be aware of his gradually changing needs and should adjust his dosage accordingly. After the initial period, the patient can begin the standarad macrobiotic way of eating. If the diabetes has arisen after the age of 35, if can be completely relieved within two to four months. However, *juvenile diabetes* is much more difficult. Many cases show initial improvement, but after reaching a certain level, for example, reducing insulin from about 60 units per day to about 10 units, they begin to fluctuate. It is very difficult to achieve a complete cure in persons who are under the age of 20.

A distant cause of juvenile diabetes is the quality of the food eaten by the mother during pregnancy. Since the diet of most people has become much worse during the past 25 years, many babies have been born with natively weak constitutions, which render them more susceptible to conditions such as diabetes. However, since they are young, juvenile diabetics should be able to regenerate their pancreatic cells more quickly than adults. The reason for their difficulty seems to be the fact that young people require more yin hormones than do adults, since they are still in the process of completing their growth. People over the age of 35 do not require so many yin hormones, since their physical structure has already had the opportunity to stabilize for a number of years.

Hyperinsulinism

This is an overly yang condition in which too much insulin is secreted. The symptoms are opposite to diabetes mellitus, and are as follows: (1) hypoglycemia (low blood sugar), (2) fatigue, (3) muscular weakness, (4) excessive perspiration and thirst, (5) nervous irritability including anxiety and neurosis, and in extreme cases, (6) convulsions and coma. If a person with this condition goes into a coma, immediate ingestion or injection of glucose will bring temporary relief.

In some cases, hyperinsulinism is brought on by an overdose of insulin. This condition is known as insulin shock. A chronic condition of hyperinsulinism may be due to tumors which involve the islets of Langerhans or to hypersensitivity of the islets to the level of blood sugar. Tumors in this area arise because of the presence of too much insulin which attracts various yin fatty acids which then coagulate.

The standard medical treatment for this condition is to remove the tumor, or in the case of hypersensitivity, to recommend a diet which is high in fat and protein and low in carbohydrate. However, this diet is similar to that recommended for diabetes, which is an opposite condition. Naturally, this does not result in a cure.

In normal circumstances, the blood sugar level remains fairly constant. Abnormal conditions are detected by means of what is known as a *glucose tolerance test*, in which a quantity of glucose, usually 100 grams, is given to the patient after a night of fasting. In a healthy person, the blood sugar level will usually not rise above 150 mg per 100 cc of blood. A person with diabetes will experience a more rapid rise in the blood sugar level, usually beyond 150 mg, and the level tends to remain above normal. Glucose may also start to appear in the urine. In the case of hyperinsulinism, the blood sugar level often falls to below 70 mg within four hours of receiving the glucose.

A person with hyperinsulinism should begin the standard macrobiotic way of eating with the following modifications: (1) Brown rice cooked with millet should comprise the principal food. Grains should not be cooked with salt. (2) Vegetables should be very lightly seasoned with oil and salt, and green leafy vegetables should be emphasized. (3) Two cups of soup may be taken daily. *Miso* or *tamari* broth soup should have a very mild taste. (4) Among beans, emphasis should be given to more yin varieties such as lentils, soybeans, and black beans. (5) On the whole, the style of cooking should be more yin.

CHAPTER EIGHT

The Nervous System

The human nervous system has two anatomical divisions: the more yang central nervous system, which includes the brain and spinal cord; and the more yin peripheral nervous system, which includes all of the nervous structures outside of the skull and vertebral canal, such as the cranio-spinal nerves and the orthosympathetic branch of the autonomic nervous system. The central nervous system acts as a "switchboard" for incoming impulses from receptors and outgoing impulses to effectors; it regulates all body activities except for chemically controlled ones, and of course is the seat for the higher conscious processes. The peripheral nervous system connects peripheral organs and tissues of the body with the central nervous system. The cranio-spinal nerves which it includes consist of the twelve pairs of cranial nerves, which are connected to the brain, and the thirty-one pairs of spinal nerves, rooted in the spinal cord. (See Fig. 54.)

The autonomic nervous system is not considered to be an anatomical division, but rather a functional unit which handles the involuntary, non-conscious body activities, such as the beating of the heart, breathing, digestive peristalsis, and so on. The autonomic system is in turn composed of two antagonistic branches, the para-sympathetic (yang) and the orthosympathetic (yin). The parasympathetic nerves have a more peripheral position of origin in the body, beginning in the brain stem and sacral region of the spinal cord (top and bottom), and passing outward through four pairs of cranial nerves and three pairs of sacral nerves. The orthosympathetic nerves have a more central position, beginning in the central section of the spine and passing outward through the corresponding spinal nerves.

In the mother's womb, all nerves in the body are actually autonomic, working automatically, but after birth, consciousness gradually emerges. That is to say, a division begins to arise between the autonomic functions and the higher, central nervous system. This division becomes most clear at the time of maturity.

In almost all organs, tissues, and smooth muscles there are pairs of autonomic nerves, one ortho- and one para-sympathetic, which act in opposite ways. Thus the whole body is held by an antagonistic yet complementary system of nervous control. Fig. 55 shows the way these nerves work in some specific body areas.

Another example of the cooperation of this two-armed system is urination. As the bladder wall contracts under parasympathetic action, the sphincter relaxes. Through orthosympathetic stimulation the opposite occurs: the bladder wall relaxes and the sphincter tightens, so that urine is retained. The parasympathetic system is especially affected by the intake of strong yin, particularly drugs and medications. Generally speaking, these items reduce the polarity between the two branches, making all body reflexes and functions less sharp. One example of a specific problem is in the uterus, where soon after drugs are begun the overstimulated parasympathetic nerves keep the uterus in a state of contraction. This situation can easily bring on a miscarriage. The same immediate effect can sometimes be observed in the

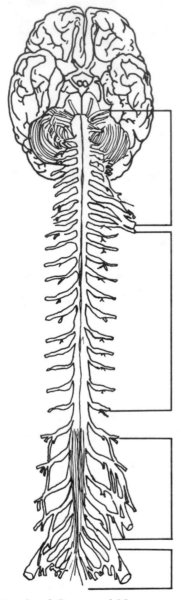

8 pairs of Cervical Nerves

12 pairs of Thoracic Nerves

5 pairs of Lumbar Nerves

5 pairs of Sacral Nerves

1 pair of Coccygeal Nerves

Fig. 54. *Branches of the spinal cord.*

eyes, where the pupils contract, and in the vascular system, where the blood vessels dilate. After continued drug use, however, the parasympathetic nerves become "worn out," yinnizing more and more; the pupils then dilate and the vessles contract.

A yang stimulus will affect the orthosympathetic system, causing the hair to "stand on end," the follicle muscles to contract, the heart to speed up, the pupils to enlarge, and the bronchi to dilate, resulting in more rapid breathing. An opposite, or yin stimulus, will affect the parasympathetic system, causing the breathing and heartbeat to slow down.

Medical researchers in Canada have found that a major problem in sickness is

	△ PARA (YANG)	▽ ORTHO (YIN)
Iris (yang)	Dilation	Constriction
Pupil (yin)	Constriction	Dilation
Blood Vessel (yang)	Vasodilation	Vasoconstriction
Cardiac Muscles (yang)	Inhibition	Stimulation
Bronchi (yin)	Constriction	Dilation
Digestive tract— wall part (yin)	Constriction	Relaxation
Digestive— sphincter (yang)	Relaxation	Constriction
Uterus—in pregnancy (yang)	Inhibition	Contraction
Hair Follicles	(none)	Constriction

Fig. 55. *Functions of the autonomic nerve.*

disharmony in the autonomic system, or in other words, poor coordination between its two branches. An absence of symptoms, however, was found not only in the case of a sensitive and balanced system, but also when the system was generally desensitized and dull. Strangely enough, following their theory in a negative way, these doctors decided to administer cortisone for certain problems, in order to dull the autonomic system, especially the parasympathetic branch. Unfortunately, cortisone has a number of unpleasant side effects. One is that long-term use often brings about slight retardation in a person. Macrobiotic treatment follows the positive side of this theory, working to sensitize and coordinate the autonomic system, producing a person who is alert and quick.

The action of the autonomic nervous system can be summed up as follows. When the parasympathetic nerves act on expanded organs, there is naturally a resultant contraction; their action on compact organs brings about expansion or dilation. The orthosympathetic nerves have a complementary, opposite effect, inhibiting the hollow organs and stimulating the compact organs. The basic principle of this action can be diagrammed as follows:

	Para (Yang)	Ortho (Yin)
Yin (hollow) organ	Yang—contract	Yin—dilate
Yang (compact) organ	Yin—dilate	Yang—contract

If you know this, you do not have to memorize long lists like the one we have been discussing; simply apply this principle to all cases.

Consciousness and Communication

To understand the manner in which the brain serves to facilitate communication, let us consider the relationships between its various components. The two major divisions of the brain are the large forebrain and the more compact small brain. Since the forebrain is more expanded, it is more yin, while the small brain is more yang. We can also divide the brain into its more central region known as the midbrain, and more peripheral region called the cortex. (See Fig. 56.)

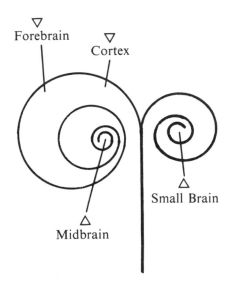

Fig. 56. *There are a number of complementary-antagonistic relationships within the spirallically formed brain and central nervous system, including the relationship between the more yang small brain and the more yin forebrain, and more yang midbrain and more yin cortex.*

Communication involves the interaction of both outgoing and incoming factors. Since impulses or messages which are dispatched are more expansive, these can be considered more yin, while those which are received are more yang. In order for communication to proceed smoothly, both of these factors need to be balanced. Within the brain, the more compacted, or central regions tend to be the areas where images and impulses are received, while outgoing communication originates in the more peripheral, or expanded areas. Among the areas shown in the diagram, the midbrain is the most central. Therefore, all nervous impulses, such as those from the eyes, ear, nose, and skin gather there. Impulses from our entire surrounding environment travel through the nervous system to this area of the brain. On the other hand, all of the images, dreams, and thought vibrations that we dispatch outward originate from the more peripheral cortex region.

When we divide the head into front and back portions, we discover that the front side is more open or expanded, while the backside is more tight and compact. In terms of receiving and dispatching, the backside receives incoming vibrations, while outgoing vibrations are dispatched from the front. Past memories, which are more yang, are generated more in the back of the brain, while more yin future images arise in the front. (See Fig. 57.)

This same difference can also be seen when we consider the relationship between the right and left hemispheres of the brain. The more yang right hemisphere is the origin of more simple or mechanical action and consciousness, while the more yin

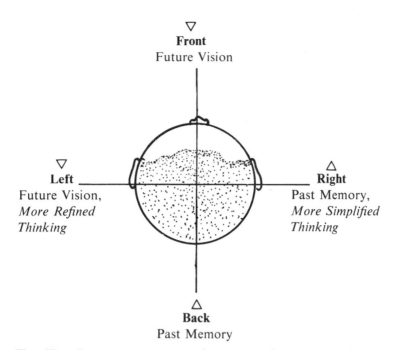

∇
Front
Future Vision

∇
Left
Future Vision,
More Refined
Thinking

△
Right
Past Memory,
More Simplified
Thinking

△
Back
Past Memory

Fig. 57. *Future vision arises in the more yin front portion of the brain, while memory arises in the more yang back section. The more yang right side is where more simplified thinking occurs, while more refined thinking arises in the more yin left side.*

left hemisphere produces more refined and complex thinking. In terms of language, more simple or basic expressions originate in the right hemisphere, while the left hemisphere creates more refined expression. Imagination, which is based mostly on futuristic thinking, develops more in the left hemisphere, while in the right hemisphere, our thinking is based more on actual past experiences.

Climatic and geographic differences throughout the world produce the tendency to develop more toward one or the other of these qualities of thinking. Therefore, in some parts of the world, people tend more toward imaginative thinking, while in others, their thinking is based more on their past experiences. Of course, each person contains both tendencies, but on the average, the general trend of a particular population will be more toward one way or the other.

Scientific thinking is based mostly on the sensorial confirmation of a particular theory or idea through controlled experimentation. This is an example of right-hemisphere thinking. On the other hand, poets, novelists, or persons with religious or spiritual inclinations base their thinking more on imagination than on experimentation, and are using the left side of their brains more. On the whole, Western civilization can be classified as a more *theoretic* culture, while various Asian countries represent more *aesthetic* cultures. The former is based more on right-side thinking, while the latter is based more on thought originating in the left side.

This relationship also corresponds to the complementary antagonism between the past and future, with the right side being more the source of past memories and the left side more of future vision.

Our modern technological civilization has arisen due to the active development of right-hemisphere thinking. This more restricted type of thinking and activity has in turn called for the proliferation of various yin types of food, such as refined sugar, chemicals, imported tropical fruits and spices, and others, as well as to the artificial synthesis of extremely expansive products like birth-control pills and LSD. Then, within many modern countries, people in the younger generations have been exposed to these types of foods from birth, and, many have taken various medications and drugs such as LSD. These extreme products have produced a rapid shift in thinking from the right side, which is predominant in modern society, towards the left side, and also from the back of the brain more toward the front. As a result, many young people started looking more toward the future, while neglecting or forgetting many previous traditions. An example is the "New Age" movement that was popular in the United States several years ago. Various modes of aesthetic expression, such as music and poetry, which result from the activation of the left hemisphere, formed an integral part of this movement.

In terms of communication, we can say that this movement emphasized the more expansive aspect of dispatching, or in other words, giving away. This can be seen in the popularity of ideas such as "love one another." In many cases, the steady intake of extreme foods has led to very unbalanced conditions where people are mostly dispatching and not receiving. When the dispatching aspect of communication becomes predominant, we call this "altruism"; while when the receiving aspect is stronger, this is known as "egocentricity." Altruism tends to develop more among those who consume a more vegetable-quality diet, while egocentricity is more the result of a diet based around animal products.

Among the branches of the autonomic nervous system, the parasympathetic branch is more active at night, while the orthosympathetic branch is more active during the day. In terms of communication, the parasympathetic system acts more as a receiver of impulses and vibrations, while dispathcing is more the function of the orthosympathetic branch.

The parasympathetic-receiver is most active during the deepest part of the night, which is between 1 and 3 A.M. It is during this time that many people have had the experience of seeing what is known as a "true dream," which means an actual perception of something that may be occurring at a great distance. As an illustration of how this process works, let us take the example of a person seeing a nighttime dream showing the death of a friend or a relative which is actually occurring at some distance. As death approaches, the person who is dying is becoming progressively more yin, meaning that the more expanded parts of the nervous system such as the orthosympathetic system and cerebral cortex become more active. These areas function more as dispatchers of outgoing images, which exist in the form of waves or vibrations. These are "caught" by the second person's parasympathetic-receiver which is more active during the evening. Therefore, he sees an image of his friend's death. The dying person can be compared to a television transmitting station which is dispatching waves in all directions, while the person who sees the dream is acting in the same manner as a television receiver which catches these waves and translates them into an image.

The entire human body is actually functioning as a complex communications machine based on the very simple code of yin and yang, or sending and receiving.

This simple code also forms the basis of the most complex computers, as well as all interactions in the universe. For example, each of our cells contains two complementary and antagonistic chemical components known as DNA and RNA. DNA is located in the central nucleus, while RNA is found more in the peripheral cytoplasm. In terms of communication, DNA functions more as the receiving component within each cell. while RNA serves more as the dispatching component. DNA can also be thought of as the repository of our past heritage, or memory, while RNA represents our future possibilities for growth.

The more yang components of the human body such as the parasympathetic system, the bones, the compacted organs, the DNA in every cell, and others, all serve as receivers of various forms of vibration, and are the repositories of our past memories. The more yin components—the orthosympathetic system, the hollow organs, RNA, and others all function as dispatchers of vibration and as the creators of our future visions.

This same relationship exists between the brain and the rest of the body. There are billions of cells compacted into the relatively small space of the brain, and each of these corresponds to one of the billions of cells existing in the expanded body. In an overall sense, we can say that the compact brain functions more as our communications receiver, while the rest of the body serves more as our communications dispatcher. In terms of time, the brain serves as the primary interpreter of past memories, while the body as a whole functions in the realization of our future dream or vision.

Our physical body is actually a compact replica of the entire universe, with the brain representing the entire past universe, and the rest of the body representing the future universe. Our universe is presently expanding in all directions, and this is replicated in our expanded body. However, the universe itself is governed by an eternal order of change in which expansion and contraction always change into one another.

In the past, the universe was contracting rather than expanding, as is reflected in the more compacted brain. As human beings, we have the capacity to extend our memory beyond the origin of this universe toward the infinite past, while our image or dream can be dispatched infinitely toward the future.

Infinity has two dimensions—infinite space and infinite time. Infinite space comprises the yin aspect of infinity, since it is constantly expanding in all directions. Infinite space is the source of all images and vibrations, and these are being continually dispatched to every galaxy, planet, and object in the universe.

The second aspect of infinity is the beginningless and endless stream of time. In comparison to space, time is yang, serving to condense or gather together all phenomena. Since we are replicas of the infinite universe, our capacity includes both of these aspects. Infinite space appears in the human consciousness as the infinite capacity for love, which is an expanding or embracing phenomenon. Infinite time manifests as our capacity for infinite memory.

Both of these capacities can be linked in the form of a cross, with infinite love representing the vertical dimension of space, and infinite memory representing the horizontal dimension of time. At the center of this figure is the human body, and these lines extend infinitely outward from there. As we continue to eat macrobiotically, our condition becomes increasingly refined, and we are not disturbed by toxins, cloudy vision, or by the rough vibrations of other people eating meat and sugar or overeating. As we become increasingly sensitive, we start to recover our infinite memory, meaning that we start to catch vibrations from infinity. At the same time, we begin to dispatch our image or dream, which exists in the form of vibration, back out toward infinity. While we are living here in the form of a human being on this tiny planet known as the earth, we begin to know what is taking place millions of light years away, as well as what occurred billions of years ago or what will occur billions of years from now. This ability is known popularly as "universal consciousness."

Universal consciousness is often thought of in terms of more sentimental expressions such as universal love, etc. Although universal consciousness includes this, it can be thought of more as the power of insight or understanding which extends beyond this solar system and galaxy, and beyond millions of galaxies and through to the dimensions of infinite space and time. These capacities do not require any special training to develop, but evolve naturally through the practice of macrobiotics. By eating small quantities of good food, chewing very well, and keeping busy, we develop our capacity to receive vibration from infinity and to dispatch vibration back to infinity. This process all depends on the quality and coordination of the body, which should ideally function as a finely-tuned instrument for receiving and dispatching infinite vibrations. This very simple method is the most universal way of developing the unlimited capacities of human consciousness.

The Macrobiotic Approach to Multiple Sclerosis and Other Diseases of the Nervous System

1.   Multiple Sclerosis (Multiple—many; Sclerosis—hardening)

Our entire body, and all of its parts, is constantly being charged with *ki* or environmental energy. This charge originates from our surroundings—the condition of the atmosphere, the motion of the earth, and the activity of celestial bodies such as stars and planets. It is this constant stream of invisible energy that actually makes life possible.

The amount and intensity of charge that we receive depends on the position of our body. For example, when we stand upright, our vertical position allows a very active energy flow up and down from the earth; this causes the heart, digestive organs, and the brain to function very actively. When we assume a horizontal position, for example when we sleep, the charge that we receive becomes less intense, and all of our bodily functions slow down.

As we saw in the section on meridian diagnosis, human life is maintained and activated by two primary forces: a centripetal force coming in to the magnetic core of the earth from stars, constellations, the sun, the moon, other celestial bodies, the atmosphere, and infinite space itself, which we call heaven's force, and a centrifugal force generated upward by the earth's rotation, which we call earth's force. Physically speaking, heaven is yin or expanded, but dynamically the force or energy which it generates is centripetal, coming in towards the earth. On the other hand, the earth is physically yang, but the energy generated by its rotation is upward and expanding.

Heaven's force enters the body through the center of the hair spiral on top of the head and exits via the sex organs. Earth's force enters through the sex organs, passes through the body and exits through the head spiral. Both of these forces run deep within the body along one central channel, and they collide at certain areas, producing an intense outward radiation of energy. The areas where this charge is most intense are the midbrain, throat, heart, stomach, and small intestines or *hara*. These five colliding places, plus the entrance and exit regions were known in India as the seven *chakras*. Heaven's downward centripetal force stronger in men, thus producing downward-extending sex organs which are external and more expanded; while earth's expanding upward force is stronger in women, resulting in sex organs which are oriented upward inside the body.

The primary, or spiritual, channel runs deep within the body slightly in front of the spine. Since the earth is rotating, the forces of heaven and earth are not straight lines but curve in a spirallic manner. In the Northern Hemisphere, heaven's force moves in a counterclockwise direction, and earth's force proceeds outward in a clockwise direction. These directions are reversed in the Southern Hemisphere. In the body, these descending helixes of energy intertwine, forming a configuration similar to the double-helix form of DNA, with one strand representing heaven's force and the other representing earth's force. In fact, the structure of DNA reflects the way in which these forces interact throughout the human body. During its course through the body, this spiral channel of energy passes through the large vein running in front of the spine, known as the *inferior vena cava*. Since this channel provides the source of our life energy, its smooth functioning is essential for our health. (See Fig. 58.)

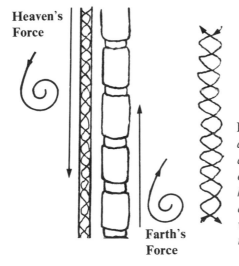

Heaven's Force

Earth's Force

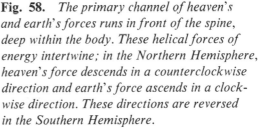

Fig. 58. *The primary channel of heaven's and earth's forces runs in front of the spine, deep within the body. These helical forces of energy intertwine; in the Northern Hemisphere, heaven's force descends in a counterclockwise direction and earth's force ascends in a clockwise direction. These directions are reversed in the Southern Hemisphere.*

This primary vertical channel activates both the right and left sides of the body with *ki* or generalized energy. The energy which animates the arms originates along this central channel in the throat and heart *chakras*. From here it branches off to the left and right. The charge of *ki* which energizes the legs originates in the *hara* region and likewise branches off to the left and right. This energy runs deep within the arms and legs, and is the cause of their motion. This charge proceeds to the center of the palms and feet, and from there, it radiates outward to the sides and toward the fingers and toes. These central regions are occasionally referred to in oriental medicine as the "heart of the hand" or the "heart of the foot." (See Fig. 59.)

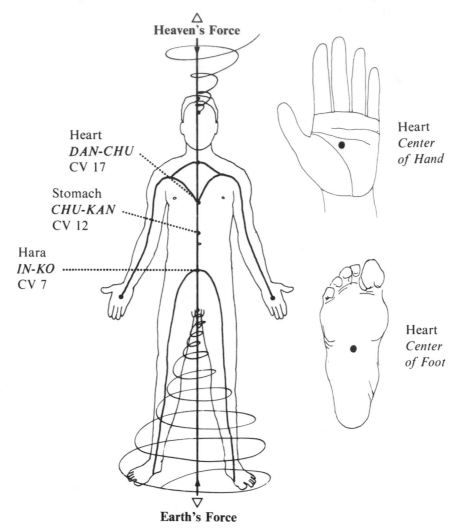

Fig. 59. *The three major regions for the generation of ki, or life energy, along the primary channel deep within the body are the heart, stomach and HARA or small intestine. Each corresponds to a point on the Conception Vessel (CV) meridian which runs upward along the front of the body. The numbers in the diagram refer to their specific locations on this meridian. The Japanese name for each point is also indicated.*

During the past 50 years, many people have been experiencing chronic weakening of this vital charge. In extreme cases, this weakening produces symptoms such as numbness and inability to move the arms and legs, organ disfunction, impaired speech, and loss of ability to think clearly. This syndrome, known as multiple sclerosis, is on the increase. Multiple sclerosis usually begins in the legs and proceeds upwards. Since this more yang part of the body is often the first region to be affected, multiple sclerosis can generally be classified as a more yin sickness. However, it can arise from continued overconsumption of both yin or yang foods, which produce the following effects:

A. Yin Cause: The vital channel becomes open and loose, resulting in a decreased conductivity for heaven's and earth's force. The majority of cases fall into this category, and result from excessive intake of sugar, fruit and fruit juice, Vitamin C, chemicals, cold beverages, medications, and other very yin substances.

B. Yang Cause: In this case, the vital channel becomes clogged with hard deposits and the flow of energy through it is impeded. The underlying cause is overconsumption of animal foods such as dairy, particularly cheese, eggs, and saturated animal fat.

In either case, the flow of energy to the arms, legs, organs, and other parts of the body diminishes, and paralysis sets in. If the legs are the first area to be affected, the charge around the *hara* region is particularly weak or stagnated, while if the arms are stricken first, the primary blockage exists around the heart and throat *chakras*.

One way of determining whether a case of multiple sclerosis is caused by excess yin or yang is to press the heart-of-the-hand point located in the center of the palm, as well as the center of the head spiral. If these regions seem unusually hard, then the M. S. is caused by too much yang. If they seem loose or soft, the cause is the opposite. The primary cause of multiple sclerosis is improper diet, but along with this, there are other factors which contribute toward its development. Let us consider these in some detail.

1. Abortion.   After an egg is fertilized and implanted, the body begins concentrating blood and *ki* energy toward the depth of the womb. This area corresponds to the *hara* region, and it is here that the intense activity of heaven's and earth's forces form the developing embryo. In the case of an abortion, the embryo is suddenly removed, and all of the centripetal forces which gather around it are dispersed throughout the body. Since the *hara* region should normally be very yang, that sudden dispersal produces a substantial weakening in this area. If this experience follows many years of poor eating, which also weakens the contracting power of this region, the result can be multiple sclerosis or weakening of the legs.

2. Appendectomy.   The yin structure—i.e., hollow, expanded—of the small and large intestines is counterbalanced by the compact appendix. So to speak, the intestines are "held together" by the appendix, in the way a fan is bound together in the center. If we suddenly remove the fan's central binding, it will collapse. In the same way, removal of the appendix causes the intestines to become loose and very weak.

The removal of the appendix increases the possibility for development of a variety of intestinal disorders such as hernia, indigestion, or bulging intestines, as well as weakening of the legs. It is also a contributing factor in the development of multiple sclerosis.

3. Removal of the ovaries.   Many women have had one or both ovaries removed in order to remove a cyst or tumor. These operations, along with hysterectomies, accelerate the development of M. S.

4. Removal of tonsils or adenoids.   The organs of the mouth correspond to the male and female sex organs in the torso. Thus, heaven's descending force creates the uvula and adenoid glands, and in the male, the penis and testis. The tongue and the tonsils are created more by earth's upward force, as are the uterus and ovaries. (See Fig. 60.) If we remove the adenoids, the effect is similar to the removal of the testis, while removing the tonsils is similar to the removal of the ovaries. These operations substantially weaken the charge of *ki* or life energy in the *hara* region, and cause the vital channel on the whole to become much weaker.

Approximately 60%–70% of all modern people have had some type of operation. About 30%–40% have had their tonsils or adenoids removed, while about 10%–15% have had their appendix removed. All of the operations mentioned above contribute toward the weakening of a person's life energy, or *ki*, especially the charge of the vital channel.

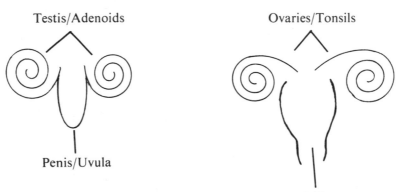

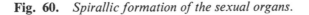

Fig. 60. *Spirallic formation of the sexual organs.*

5. *Long hot baths or showers.* Many people take a 20-minute hot bath or shower every day. Only one generation ago, this practice was not so common. People either showered quickly or washed themselves with a wet sponge or towel, and bathed about once a week. Long hot baths or showers cause us to lose minerals, which are needed in order to maintain an active charge of heaven's and earth's force along the vital channel.

6. *Loss of natural contact.* Most of us in modern society always wear shoes when we go outside. For those of us who live in cities, we usually walk only on sidewalks or streets made of asphalt or concrete. Our feet never come in direct contact with the earth. Our modern environment serves to block the energy of heaven and earth. We further isolate ourselves from this energy by wearing nylon stockings, synthetic socks, and other artificially-produced clothing, or by using artificical rugs, curtains, furniture, blankets, and other unnatural items in our homes.

All of these factors—operations, unnatural life styles, artificial environments— combined with our modern way of eating, have produced a weaker-quality human being known as modern man.

To diagnose whether someone is prone toward multiple sclerosis, push the point located in the center of the throat just above the top of the breast bone. Pain in this area means that mucus and fat deposits have started to form in the throat, and that the spiritual channel is somewhat blocked in this area. This congestion is often followed by blockage around the heart region.

The macrobiotic approach to this disease centers on revitalizing the patient's charge of life energy by dissolving stagnation, particularly along the spiritual channel. Our treatment includes three aspects: (1) dietary adjustment, (2) modification of lifestyle, and in some cases, (3) external applications or treatments.

C.   Dietary Suggestions for the Relief of Multiple Sclerosis.   To relieve yin M.S., a person should begin following the standard macrobiotic diet, with the following modifications, while a person with yang M.S. should observe a diet similar to that far more yang type of cancer.

1.   All food should be of vegetable quality.
2.   Whole grains should comprise as much as 60%–70% of the daily diet. Grains should be eaten primarily in their whole form (e.g., brown rice, millet, kasha) rather than as flour. However, among flour products, whole buckwheat noodles (*soba*) may be eaten on occasion. Yeasted breads should be strictly avoided.
3.   *Gomasio* should be more yang, perhaps 10:1. If the patient can tolerate it, 9:1 or 8:1 *gomasio* can be used.
4.   *Miso* or *tamari* broth soups should be somewhat thicker than usual. However, if the patient becomes thirsty, decrease the amount of these seasonings.
5.   Oil should be used sparingly, and only in cooking.
6.   Among vegetables, the patient should eat about 1/2 root vegetables and about 1/2 hard, leafy green vegetables. Vegetables should be cooked slowly over a low flame. The *nishime*, or waterless, cooking style is also highly advisable. Several varieties of root vegetables can be combined with *kombu* and cooked in this manner. This dish should be seasoned with *tamari* or *miso*.
7.   Raw salad should be avoided. Instead, the patient may occasionally have some boiled salad, in which the vegetables are only lightly boiled for one or two minutes.
8.   Beans and seaweeds should be eaten every day; however, the percentage of beans should not exceed 10%.
9.   Fruit or fruit desserts should be strictly avoided.
10.   Animal food should be avoided. However, if the patient experiences cravings, vegetable-protein dishes such as *seitan* may be used. If the cravings are not satisfied by this, the patient may occasionally have a small quantity of little dried fish.
11.   Tea and other standard beverages should be used only when the person is thirsty.

D.   Modifications in Lifestyle.
1.   Long hot baths or showers should be avoided. A person with this condition should also not go swimming in a chlorinated swimming pool, or for more than several minutes in a freshwater lake or stream. However, the patient may swim in the ocean.
2.   Synthetic clothing, especially underwear, stockings, and socks, should not be used.
3.   Wigs or hairpieces should not be worn.
4.   A person with this condition should not wear shoes or socks while indoors, and should often go walking barefoot on grass or soil.

E. External Treatments.   The following treatments are aimed at helping to dissolve energy blockages and stimulate the charge of *ki* along the spiritual channel.

1. Treatment of the Back.   In cases where the legs are affected, energy blockages along the primary spiritual channel occur principally around the *hara* region, and if the arms are paralyzed, around the heart and throat regions. To comprehensively treat these blockages, we can apply heat to the regions of the spine corresponding to the three main body *chakras*—the heart, stomach, and *hara*. If you press the spine in these areas, a person with multiple sclerosis will usually experience pain. (See Fig. 61.)

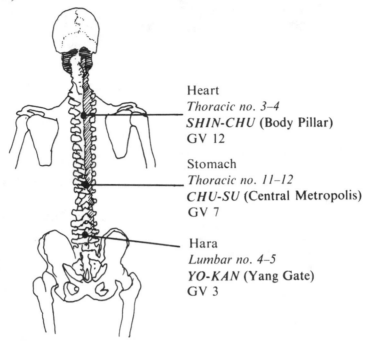

Heart
Thoracic no. 3–4
SHIN-CHU (Body Pillar)
GV 12

Stomach
Thoracic no. 11–12
CHU-SU (Central Metropolis)
GV 7

Hara
Lumbar no. 4–5
YO-KAN (Yang Gate)
GV 3

Fig. 61.   *The three major points on the spine which correspond to the three major body* chakras *are indicated in the above diagram with their Japanese names and translations. These points can be found in the spaces between the vertebrae, and their locations are noted above, along with the corresponding location of each point on the Govering Vessel (GV) meridian which runs up along the center of the spine.*

Either cigarette moxa or direct moxa can be used to generate heat on these points. When applying cigarette moxa, use the technique described in the chapter, *The Way of Diagnosis.* If you have real moxa, it can be applied directly to these points for the same purpose.

Along with these points, we may also need to treat other regions of the spine, all of which lie on the *governing vessel* meridian which runs along the entire spine. These points can be determined by pressing along the entire spine with your thumbs inserted in between the vertebrae. Moxa can then be applied to the regions where pain is felt.

After treating the specific regions described above, cigarette moxa should be applied along the entire length of the spine. For yin M. S., hold the cigarette about

1/4 inch from the spine, starting at the top, and slowly move it downward toward the base. Start at the bottom of the spine and move upward for yang M. S. If you aren't sure whether the disease is more yin or yang, start at the bottom and move upward.

The *bladder meridian* runs down the back on either side of the spine. There are several important points on this meridian which are effective in treating multiple sclerosis. Moxa can be applied to bladder points 31–34 which are located on the lower back, or to bladder points 35, 40, and 60, which are located on the back of both legs.

A treatment such as this should be administered about once a week. It may take about 15–20 minutes to treat all of these points. In some cases, patients who have been confined to a wheelchair may actually be able to stand up after only one treatment. However, if this method is not combined with a proper diet, the spiritual channel will soon become blocked, and the patient's condition will again worsen.

The spine can also be treated with a hot ginger towel. Prepare hot ginger water in the same way as for a ginger compress. Instead of applying the towel to only one area, rub the entire spine with it until the skin turns very red.

2. Treatment of the Hands and Feet. A person who has multiple sclerosis should soak both feet every night in hot water. While the feet are soaking, scrub them briskly with a towel, with particular attention to the toes. This massage will stimulate the meridians which begin or end at the toes. Several times each day, rub some grated ginger into the heart of the hand and heart of the foot points. This practice will also help to stimulate the patient's *ki* flow.

3. Chanting. Chanting vibrates the spiritual channel and helps to dissolve hardening. It should therefore be practiced every day. Sit in a straight position and breathe deeply. After a minute or so, begin to utter the sound of AUM or SU. Chanting is especially helpful if repeated frequently.

When combined with proper food, these methods can bring about a cure in three to four, or at the utmost, six months. This approach involves no danger or side effects, and is the most sure and fundamental way of solving this problem.

2. Parkinson's Disease

The symptom of this illness is an uncontrolable shaking. There are two types: (1) yang Parkinson's disease, which manifests itself as a large or very quick shaking motion, and (2) yin Parkinson's disease, which appears as a slower or less active motion. The first type is caused by the overconsumption of foods like meat, eggs, and other animal products, while the second results from the overconsumption of yin. A person with either type should stop the intake of both extremes and begin the standard macrobiotic way of eating. As a supplemental treatment, a hot ginger towel can be applied to the spine in the same way as for multiple sclerosis. This can be repeated daily. Parkinson's disease can be relieved in anywhere from one to six months.

3. Epilepsy

Epilepsy is a yin sickness. It is similar to the experiencing of a dull, heavy pressure in the head after drinking too much beer or other beverage. Epilepsy results from the overexpansion of the cells of the brain. When the brain tissue becomes over-expanded, it pinches the intricate network of nerve cells within the brain to the point where their nervous impulses are temporarily cut off. The person then becomes un-conscious and this loss of functioning ability is known as an epileptic seizure.

Seizures occur more frequently at night, during humid weather, or during the full moon. (The yang brightness of the full moon causes fluid to be attracted upward toward the head.) Seizures also occur frequently after parties or social occasions at which much liquid has been consumed. Men are more prone to epilepsy, since they tend to consume more fluid than women. Among women, those who have taken birth control pills have a higher incidence of epilepsy than those who have not.

Headaches or pressure in the head indicate a tendency toward epilepsy. This is especially true in the case of migraine headaches, which can be considered as a begin-ning stage of this disease. If you experience dizziness when you suddenly stand up, you are also beginning to develop epilepsy. The number of people who have what we might term a "preepileptic" condition is very large, perhaps as many as 50% of the total population.

A person with epilepsy usually knows when a seizure is about to happen. If such a warning is perceived, in order to offset or minimize the severity of the attack, an *umeboshi* plum, *tekka*, or *gomasio* should be eaten several times at intervals of 5–10 minutes. Therefore, a person with epilepsy should carry one of these condi-ments at all times.

The major cause of epilepsy is the repeated overconsumption of liquid. In order to relieve epilepsy, the intake of liquid should be strictly controlled, and sugar should be avoided entirely, since it changes into water in the body. Within the standard macrobiotic way of eating, more yang food items such as root vegetables should be emphasized, and our method of cooking should be slightly more yang. Also, fruit should be avoided, as should beverages like beer, wine, other alcoholic drinks, milk, soda, fruit juice, and others. The following sad case illustrates the importance of controlling liquid in dealing with epilepsy.

More than ten years ago a young man in his early twenties began macrobiotics after having suffered epileptic seizures for nearly seven years. He had been taking medication to control the seizures, and was able to eliminate it after two months. His seizures stopped completely after the third month. Naturally he became much more happy and active. He went to a summer camp about six months later, and while he was there I received a telegram stating that he had died. It seemed that the weather had been very hot, so one night he had gone into town with friends and had three cans of beer. Following this, he took beer back to the camp and drank several more cans before going to sleep. He got up the next morning at 5:00, went to the lake for a swim, and had a seizure while swimming.

There are several things that can be done to minimize the effect of an epileptic seizure. When a seizure arises, place a small piece of wood, such as a spatula or chopstick, between the patient's teeth to prevent him from biting his tongue. To reduce expansion of the brain cells, apply a cold towel to the forehead and to the back of the neck, as well as to the hands and feet. Also, apply continual deep pressure to the points indicated in Fig. 62 on both large toes. These measures can reduce to about three minutes a seizure which would normally last ten minutes.

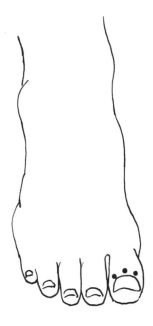

Fig. 62. *Specific pressure points to be used in the treatment of epileptic seizures.*

CHAPTER NINE

The Reproductive System

The Male Reproductive System

The *testes*, located below the torso in the sac called the *scrotum*, are the primary male organs of reproduction. The peripheral layer of the testes, called the *tunica albuginea*, contains about 250 *lobules* or chambers. Each chamber holds from one to three minute *seminiferous tubules*, in which sperm are formed. (See Fig. 63.)

Mature spermatozoa lie on the inner surface of each tubule, with their heads imbedded in the inner lining and their tails facing outwards. (See Fig. 63.) Sperm are created through a process of yinnization in which the cells of the tubules differentiate into millions of sperm. Sperm are eventually discharged from each tubule, floating upwards through the *rete testis* and *efferent ducts* to a region known as the *epididymis*. From here, sperm must flow downward, a difficult direction for yin to move. This process is slow and results in a temporary accumulation in the epididymis. Sperm may be stored in this region for weeks, months, or even years.

Ejaculation of the seminal fluid occurs as a result of contractions of the lower bladder muscles and the smooth muscle of the prostate gland, along with contraction of the muscles in the excretory ducts, especially the *ductus deferens*. These contractions enable the sperm to move quickly, and an average ejaculation contains about 200 to 400 million sperm. If sperm do not enter the uterus, they soon die as a result of oxidation, but if they do, they can live for about three to five days. Their ability to fertilize an egg, however, is limited to about 24 hours.

Diseases of the Male Reproductive System

1. Inability to Produce Sperm

The production of sperm through the yin process of differentiation requires a more yang quality blood. Men who cannot create sperm usually have a very weak quality of blood, and often have a tendency toward anemia, and in extreme cases, are susceptible to leukemia. This results from the overconsumption of yin foods, and can be overcome through the standard macrobiotic way of eating, with emphasis on the type of foods recommended for anemia.

2. Impotency

Impotency means the inability to achieve an erection, which is made possible by the contraction of muscles around the bladder. This condition usually arises when these muscles become loose and expanded, and lose their normal contracting power. This condition is generally caused by too many expansive foods, and can be relieved through the standard way of eating, with emphasis on more compacted grains such as buckwheat, as well as root vegetables like carrots and burdock.

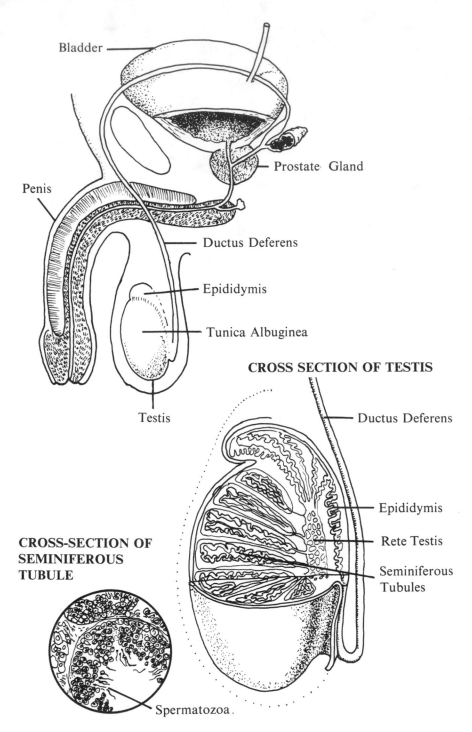

Fig. 63. *The Male Reproductive System.*

3.   Blockage of the Semen Ducts

This arises in the same way as hardening of the arteries, and is caused by the overconsumption of animal foods like eggs, meat, and dairy products, all of which contain saturated fat, as well as by foods like sugar and fruits which produce fat and mucus. Blockage can be relieved through the standard way of eating, along with limiting the use of oil and a temporary avoidance of nuts and other oily foods.

4. Hydrocele

This is an accumulation of water around or in the testis, and is caused by the excessive intake of more expansive foods, particularly fluid. This condition can be overcome through the standard way of eating, and by controlling the intake of liquid.

The Female Reproductive System

1. The Ovaries

The ovaries are the primary organs of the female reproductive system. Each of these tiny paired organs is about the size of an almond, and it is here that the production of eggs takes place. The central region of the ovaries is known as the *medulla*, while the outer layer is called the *cortex*. The medulla contains blood and lymphatic vessels and smooth muscle fibers, while the cortex contains *follicles* in various stages of development. The outer surface of the ovary is covered by a single layer of cells called the *germinal epithelium*. (See Fig. 64.)

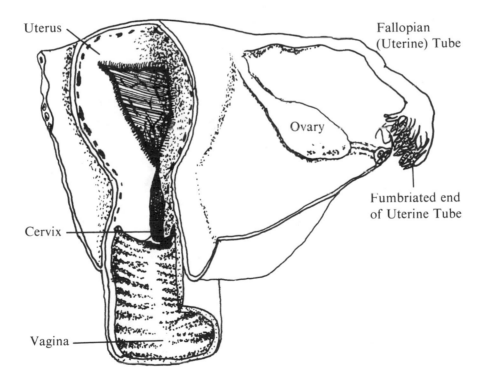

Fig. 64. *The Female Reproductive System.*

A follicle consists of an ovum surrounded by one or several layers of *follicle cells.* (See Fig. 65.) At birth, the ovaries contain about 800,000 follicles. This number decreases until, at menopause, few, if any, follicles remain. Mature women have about 400,000 follicles in their ovaries. The decrease in the number of follicles is brought about (1) by their use in the creation of ova and (2) by a process called *atresia* whereby they degenerate and are discharged from the body during menstruation.

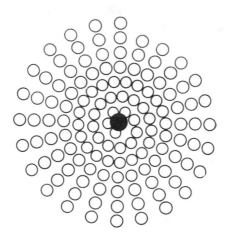

Fig. 65. *Schematic representation of follicle. Within each follicle, the follicle cells which surround the developing ovum are arranged in a spiral pattern. The egg is created by a process of contraction, or yangization.*

As an ovum matures, the follicle cells surrounding it expand and increase in number, and irregular spaces appear between the cells. These spaces are filled with a liquid called *follicular fluid.* The follicle cells which surround the ovum arrange themselves in a spiral pattern. The egg lies at the center of this spiral, and is formed by a process of contraction, or yangization, which is the opposite of the process by which sperm are created. When a follicle has reached maturity, it will either rupture and release its ovum, or collapse and decompose. The former process is known as ovulation.

2. Ovulation

About 400 of the approximately 800,000 follicles present at birth mature and discharge ova, while the remainder decompose. On the average, three to five of these 400 mature follicles undergo fertilization and eventual development into a human being.

Following ovulation, the egg, which is yang, enters the *fimbriated*, or finger-like end of the Fallopian tube, and begins its downward, yang movement. At this stage, two possibilities exist:

1. If intercourse has taken place, the egg has the possibility of being fertilized. The union of egg and sperm occurs in the fimbriated end of the uterine tube. Since sperm cells are yin, they begin an upward course after entering the vagina. If an ovum is fertilized, it begins to develop as it passes through the uterine tube and into the uterus. Implantation of the fertilized ovum in the uterus takes place after about 7–10 days.

If the path of the fertilized ovum is blocked, it will often implant in the Fallopian tube. This condition is known as tubal pregnancy, and usually results in the rupture of the Fallopian tube due to the growth of the embryo. The resulting hemorrhage may have very serious effects, and in some cases, can lead to death. Tubal pregnancies usually arise when the Fallopian tubes are blocked by thick deposits of mucus or fat, and the major causes of this are foods which contain saturated fat. This condition can also arise if the fertilized ovum does not move through the Fallopian tube quickly enough on its way to the uterus, resulting from the overconsumption of sugar, spices, tropical fruits, and other similarly extreme foods.

The uterus averages $2\frac{1}{2}$ inches in length and weighs approximately 50 grams. It has a capacity of 2 cc to 5 cc, and is tightly constructed. During pregnancy, it increases substantially, and at full term reaches a length of about 20 inches, a weight of about 1,000 gm, and a capacity of between 5,000 cc and 7,000 cc. The uterus returns to its original condition following delivery.

2.   If sperm are not present at the time of ovulation, the ovum disintegrates in its passage through the uterine tube, and is discharged through the process of menstruation.

3.   Menstruation

The 28-day cycle of menstruation correlates with the process of ovulation, and the length of time taken for each stage in this cycle is largely dependent on the types of food that a woman eats. (See Fig. 66.) For example, if a woman is eating primarily cooked whole grains and vegetables, menstruation should take only three days, as compared to the five days usually necessary for a woman who is eating a diet high in meat, sugar, and dairy products. The next phase, in which the uterine lining regenerates itself, usually takes two days. However, with proper eating this can be accomplished in a single day. The following stage, in which the follicle matures, lasts about eight days, and ovulation should occur in the part of the cycle which is exactly opposite to the onset of menstruation. Ovulation is followed by the premenstrual or *progravid* phase, during which a structure known as the *corpus luteum* develops within the ruptured follicle. During this phase, the corpus luteum matures and secretes *progesterone*, a hormone that influences the changes that take place in the uterine wall during the second half of the menstrual cycle. The follicle and corpus luteum eventually decompose during this phase, and are discharged during menstruation.

If a woman is eating properly, her menstrual cycle should correlate with the monthly lunar cycle. During the full moon, the atmosphere becomes brighter, or yang. A more yang girl will menstruate at this time, since the condition of the atmosphere will cause her to become excessively yang, thus necessitating the discharge of this excess. During the new moon, the atmosphere becomes yin, and a yin woman will usually menstruate in response to this influence. If, when a woman begins to eat properly, she menstruates in between the full and the new moon, this is an indication that her condition is also "in-between." However, the onset of menstruation will gradually start to coincide with either of these times.

During the menstrual period, a woman's excess is discharged through the skin as well as through the menstrual flow. A woman should not wash her hair or take a shower during this time, since both of these tend to draw this excess away from its normal course of discharge. When this happens, a woman's face may easily become flushed, and she may often become upset.

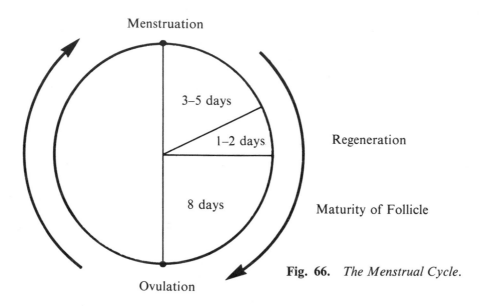

Fig. 66. *The Menstrual Cycle.*

Diseases of the Female Reproductive System

1. Menstrual Disorders

A. Menstrual Cramps. Cramps are usually caused by an excessive intake of animal products like meat, fish, eggs, and dairy food, in combination with too many expansive foods. To relieve menstrual cramps, stop these extremes and begin the standard macrobiotic way of eating. They will disappear in two to three months. This condition can be diagnosed by observing the area between the upper lip and the nose. If a horizontal line or ridge appears in this area when a woman smiles, she is most likely suffering from menstrual cramps.

B. Excessive Menstrual Flow. This can result from either an excessive intake of overly-yin or overly-yang foods. In the case of too many contractive foods, the blood thickens and the flow lasts longer. This is often accompanied by an unpleasant odor. When too many expansive foods are consumed, the blood becomes thinner than normal, and menstruation is prolonged. When a woman eats a more balanced or central diet, menstruation will be of shorter duration than what is common today, and the flow will be light.

C. Irregular Menstrual Cycle.   If the menstrual cycle is too short, totalling only 24 instead of 28 days, for instance, this usually indicates an overly-yang condition. If the cycle is longer than average, lasting from 32 to 35 days, this usually means that a woman is too yin. Both conditions can be corrected by eating a more balanced or central diet.

2. Anteversion (Retroversion) of the Uterus

In this condition, the uterus is abnormally tilted either slightly toward the front or toward the back. In many cases, it returns to its normal position after a woman becomes pregnant. If the uterus leans forward, the cause is too much yang, and if it tilts towards the back, it is caused by an excess of yin. This condition can be relieved through the standard way of eating, with slight modifications depending on the direction in which the uterus is slanted.

3. Vaginal Discharge

As we discussed in the chapter, *The Progressive Development of Sickness*, deposits of fat and mucus often accumulate in the uterus, Fallopian tubes, and in and around the ovaries. Uterine deposits usually produce vaginal discharge. If this discharge is yellowish in color, a cyst may be developing, while a white discharge is less serious, but can lead to the development of a "soft" type of cyst. A green discharge may indicate cancer, particularly if it has been occurring for any length of time. Vaginal discharges may be accompanied by an odor. The macrobiotic approach to this problem is discussed below as well as in the chapter, *The Progressive Development of Sickness*.

4. Uterine and Ovarian Cysts

As we saw in the chapter, *The Progressive Development of Sickness*, the solidification of mucus or fat around the ovaries often results in an ovarian cyst, while if it occurs within the uterus, especially in the cervical area, a uterine cyst is created. The over-consumption of foods which create fat and mucus such as dairy products, sugar, fruit and fruit juices, nut butters, oily foods, and animal fats all contribute to the development of cysts. Naturally, these items should be eliminated, and the standard macrobiotic way of eating adopted in order to relieve these conditions.

A hot ginger compress should be applied every day to the area of the womb and ovaries in cases where a cyst or tumor is blocking the Fallopian tubes. This should be continued for 10 to 14 days in conjunction with the standard diet.

The ginger compress is not necessary in cases of vaginal discharges that are not accompanied by a cyst or tumor. One of the most effective treatments for relieving a vaginal discharge is a hot hip bath. Ideally, the bath water should contain dried leafy greens such as *daikon* or turnip greens. To prepare this bath, hang about 50 bunches of these leaves to dry, either near a window or outside. The leaves will first turn yellow and then brown, at which time they are suitable for use. Boil two or three bunches of dried leaves for 10–20 minutes in several quarts of water, to which sea salt or *kombu* seaweed can be added. The water will turn brownish in color. Then, run hot water in the bath tub, add the mixture along with another handful of sea salt, and get in. Cover your upper body with a thick towel to avoid chills and to absorb perspiration. As the water begins to cool, add more hot water, and stay in the tub for 10–15 minutes.

During this time, your lower body will become very red as circulation in the area increases, and the stagnated fat and mucus inside the vagina will start to loosen. Immediately following the bath, douche with a preparation made with a pinch of sea salt, the juice of ½ lemon, and *bancha* tea. This will help to dislodge the deposits of mucus and fat, which have been loosened by the bath. Continue this procedure for five days to two weeks, depending on the severity of the condition. During this time, you should eat very well and especially avoid all dairy products, since these are the primary cause of accumulations which develop in the female sex organs.

If dried leaves are not available, add several handfuls of sea salt to the bath water instead. Hip baths, together with ginger compresses, are effective for any type of cysts or tumor in the female sex organs.

A special tampon preparation can also be used to help relieve vaginal discharges. Mix one part sesame oil with two parts grated ginger, add a pinch of sea salt, and coat a cotton tampon with the mixture. Insert as you would insert a regular tampon and leave in for about one hour. After removal, douche with the *bancha* tea mixture described above. If the ginger causes irritation, reduce the amount and then gradually increase it with each application. This should be repeated once a day for three or four days.

Most cysts are soft when they begin to form, but with the continuation of an improper diet, they harden and often calcify. This type of cyst is something like a stone, and is very difficult to dissolve. Some varieties of cysts contain fat and protein, and may even begin to form skin, hair, and calcium deposits resembling teeth. These are called *dermoid cysts*, and are the result of eating the foods mentioned above. Oral contraceptives also contribute to cyst formation.

5. Vaginismus

This is a spasm of the vaginal muscles. It may arise during intercourse, and is similar to cramps that arise in the legs. The cause is excess yin. This condition can be remedied through the standard diet, while salt, *umeboshi*, or *gomasio* will help to relieve the muscle spasm.

6. Prolapsed Uterus

This condition develops when the uterus drops, and part of it begins to protrude into the vagina. An excessive intake of yin foods causes this problem by weakening the muscles and other structures which normally hold the uterus in place. The standard macrobiotic way of eating will reverse this condition.

Venereal Diseases

There are three types of venereal disease:

1. Chancroid

The infecting agent in this illness is a bacteria known as *hemophilus ducreyi.* ·Contact with this bacteria may result in the appearance of multiple soft lesions, or "chancres," in the genital area, often accompanied by swollen lymph nodes.

2. Gonorrhea

This inflammatory condition of the mucus membranes in the reproductive organs is caused by a gonococcus, *Neisseria gonorrhoeae*, and symptoms usually occur within several days after contact.

3. Syphilis

This chronic illness is caused by a spirochete, *Treponema pallidum.* Symptoms appear in three stages. In the *primary stage*, a lesion which gradually develops into a hard chancre, appears on the sex organs two to four weeks after contact. Then, the chancre often disappears, leaving the impression that the sickness is cured.

In the *secondary stage*, symptoms appear 6 to 18 weeks after contact, and because the bacteria have spread through the bloodstream, may involve almost any organ in the body. Since the body tries to discharge the infection towards the outside, skin manifestations are common, and the symptoms of this stage are often confused with other illnesses.

The symptoms of the *tertiary stage* appear six months to several years after contact, and involve the decomposition or structural degeneration of areas such as the bones, the walls of the blood vessels, or the brain. This may also occur in any of the organs, and eventually leads to death.

Venereal disease most easily affects (1) those who consume large quantities of animal products including dairy, and (2) those who regularly consume large quantities of very yin foods like alcohol, sugar, and drugs. A person who eats cooked grains and vegetables is much less susceptible. Features such as a milky or cheesey complexion, red spots on the face from the consumption of fruit and sugar, or a nose or fingers that show a reddish or purple color, may indicate the impure blood condition that can lead to venereal disease. A person with these disorders often gives the impression of being unclean.

To relieve venereal disease, the following dietary practices should be observed, for the purpose of purifying the blood and eliminating the bacteria:
1. Only vegetable foods should be eaten, with the exception of an occasional side-dish of a very yin fish such as carp.
2. Fruits, salad, and other yin foods should be completely avoided, as should any food that produces an acidic blood condition.
3. The principal food should be unrefined cereal grains. Secondary foods

should include vegetables which are adequately seasoned with salt and oil; condiments like *gomasio* and *tekka*; *kinpira* (root vegetables such as burdock and carrots cut into matchstick pieces or slivered, sautéed with a small amount of oil and water, and cooked until the water evaporates); *shiokombu* (*kombu* seaweed pickled in *tamari*); *azuki* beans cooked with *kombu*; *hijiki* and other seaweeds which are cooked with *tamari* and oil; strong *miso* soup which can include scallions and dumplings made from sweet brown rice; *koi-koku* (a stew made with a whole carp, burdock, and *miso*); as well as pickles which are processed in salt, rice bran, or *miso*.

4. Recommended beverages include roasted grain tea (rice or barley) which is boiled with a pinch of salt; brown rice soup; and *azuki* bean and *kombu* drink (made by boiling these together with a pinch of salt and extracting the juice). As many as seven cups of these beverages may be consumed daily in order to relieve thirst.

This more restricted way of eating should be observed for one or two months, even in cases where the disease has been medically treated, to establish a healthy blood quality and ensure the elimination of the disease. The standard macrobiotic way of eating can be resumed after this period.

CHAPTER TEN

The Face and Head

The Macrobiotic Approach to Eye Diseases

1. Detachment of the Retina

Light entering the eyes normally focuses on the retina, where it creates an image that is transferred to the brain by the optic nerve. The retina is a sensitive membrane containing nerve endings, and is attached to the rear wall of the eyeball. (See Fig. 67.) Under certain circumstances, however, it starts to detach or separate. When this happens, light no longer focuses on the retina, and blindness often results. Separation or detachment is a yin characteristic, and this problem results from the overconsumption of more expansive foods, particularly liquids. To understand this process, paste two pieces of paper together and put them in water. They will soon begin to separate. The only cure for a detached retina is a very delicate operation. But since an operation does not eliminate the cause, the retina will often detach again after several years.

To relieve this problem, one should observe the standard macrobiotic way of eating, along with the following modifications: (1) control the intake of liquids; (2) control the intake of fruit; (3) avoid sugar entirely, since it changes into water in the body; (4) avoid raw vegetables; (5) avoid alcoholic beverages and fruit juice; (6) avoid watery cooking. These suggestions are aimed at reducing the body's excessive water accumulation, which is responsible for the detached retina. As the body dries, the retina will begin to reattach itself, and sight will gradually return.

Once I met with a man who was suffering from this problem. His condition did not improve even after he had begun to eat macrobiotically. I learned that the only type of oil he had been using was corn oil. When he substituted the more yang, roasted sesame oil, his eyesight returned in five days. Sesame oil was traditionally used to treat a wide variety of eye troubles. Since oil is yin, it repels excess water, which is also yin. For medicinal use, heat a small amount of sesame oil and pour it through a piece of sanitized cotton. Store this strained oil in a small jar and apply one or two drops directly to the eyes with an eyedropper. This can be continued once a day until the eye problem clears up.

2. Cataracts

With this condition, a milky film, which blocks the passage of light, develops in the crystalline lens of the eye or its capsule, and can eventually cause blindness. Cataracts develop over a long period of time, and are generally caused by expansive foods such as coffee, sugar, citrus fruit, strong drugs, dairy products, and others. Cataracts also form, however, when the gelatinous lens is composed of saturated animal fat resulting from the intake of meat and eggs, as well as cheese, butter, and other dairy foods.

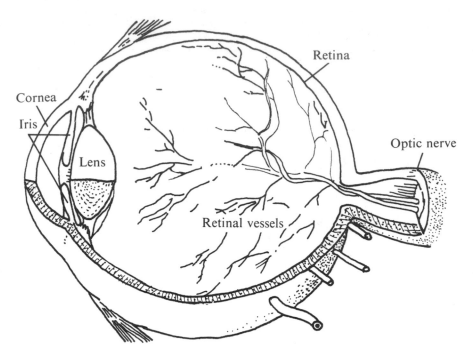

Fig. 67. *Cross-section of the human eye.*

To relieve this condition, (1) avoid the above foods and begin the standard macro-biotic way of eating; (2) apply hot water or warm *bancha* tea compresses to the eyes five or six times a day; (3) apply one or two drops of strained sesame oil to the eyes every day before going to bed in order to speed the discharge of yin. Cataracts can be relieved in about three or four months with this approach.

3. Glaucoma

Glaucoma occurs when the fluid in the eyeball begins to exert abnormal pressure against the other regions of the eye. This pressure, caused by excessive liquid intake, may damage the retina and destroy portions of the optic nerve, and often results in blindness. Draining this liquid is a standard medical treatment, but, because the cause is ignored, this condition often returns after several weeks or months. Along with the overconsumption of liquid, glaucoma can be caused by the intake of other expansive foods such as sugar, milk, and fruit. Diabetes often accompanies this condition, since both are caused by similar types of food. The macrobiotic approach to glaucoma is basically the same as that for cataracts.

About 12 years ago I met a minister suffering from glaucoma. He was judged to be legally blind. One night he dreamed that he had recovered his sight. The following day, he met a woman who told him about macrobiotics. He later came to see me with his wife assisting him, and they both began to practice macrobiotics. To relieve his condition, the strict control of liquid was essential. After several months, he again visited with his wife, and I advised him to increase the amount of soup that he was having and to add more green vegetables, since he had become very thin and dry.

Two weeks later he came for a surprise visit without his wife. His sight was returning. He then visited every other day, and after ten days he was able to go out without his cane. He had been cured. He was in his seventies and was a very humble man. He had been able to control himself to the extent of being able to overcome his problem.

4. Nearsightendness

In this case, the light entering the lens focuses in front of, rather than on, the retina. (See Fig. 68.) This condition can result from either of two basic causes. The first type occurs when the eyeball elongates as a result of the overconsumption of expansive, or yin foods, although the lens itself doesn't change. About 95% of all present cases of nearsightedness result from this cause. In the second type, the eyeball stays the same but the lens contracts. This is caused by the overconsumption of yang foods such as meat and salt.

To relieve the first type of nearsightedness, begin the standard macrobiotic way of eating, while controlling the intake of yin, including liquid. The second type of nearsightedness can be treated by the standard way of eating with a slight emphasis toward good quality yin foods and a more yin style of preparation. In both conditions, improvement will occur gradually.

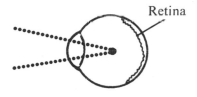

Fig. 68. *Nearsightedness.*

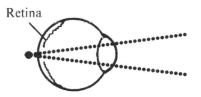

Fig. 69. *Farsightedness.*

5. Farsightendness

When the eyeball is smaller or more contracted than usual, light will focus at a point behind the retina causing farsightedness. (See Fig. 69.) Since babies have smaller eyeballs, during their first five months to one year they normally have this condition. Many elderly people are farsighted because, with age, the eyeball starts to shrink. To relieve this more yang condition, meat and other animal products should be avoided, and salt should be used in moderation. The standard macrobiotic way of eating should be adopted, and more oil than usual can be used in cooking.

6. Crossed Eyes

There are three basic causes of crossed eyes. (See Fig. 70.) The first type, in which the eyes point inward towards the nose, results from the overconsumption of foods such as eggs, meat, or salt. To relieve this condition, observe the standard macrobiotic way of eating with less salt and very little or no animal food. The second type, in which the eyes point outward, is caused more by expansive foods. Observing the

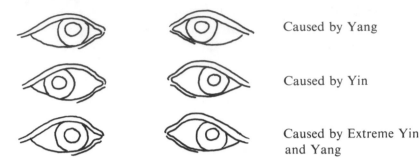

Caused by Yang

Caused by Yin

Caused by Extreme Yin
and Yang

Fig. 70. *Crossed eyes.*

standard way of eating along with controlling the intake of yin, will help this problem. The third type, in which one eye points inward and the other points outward, results from extremes of both yin and yang in one's diet, and can be relieved by eating foods which are more central or balanced.

7. Color Blindness

There are two basic types of color blindness. One is caused by the overconsumption of meat, salt, and animal foods. With this condition, a person is insensitive to the color red, which is yang. The second type is caused by too many yin foods, and results in an inability to detect colors at the opposite, or blue-green end of the spectrum. In both cases, a person should observe the standard macrobiotic way of eating. With yang color blindness, the person should moderate his use of salt and avoid most animal foods, while emphasizing items which are slightly more yin. For the opposite type of color blindness, a slightly more yang selection and preparation of foods should be emphasized.

The eyes are closely related to the liver and the sexual organs. When dealing with eye troubles, the most important factor is proper diet, along with various applications such as sesame oil drops. At the same time, we should always consider their relationship to the liver, and use such applications as hot ginger compresses to treat this organ. Simple eye exercises are also helpful. For example, close your eyes and cover them with your palms. Move them up and down, then left and right, and then rotate them in a clockwise and then in a counterclockwise direction. Repeat each motion about thirty times before moving on to the next.

In the chapter, *The Way of Diagnosis*, we outlined the major pressure-points useful in diagnosing and treating eye problems. Simple massage or cigarette moxa can be applied to these points to help relieve any type of eye disorder. Eye problems are often accompanied by tension on the sides of the head as well as in the back of the neck. Simple light massage will release tension and accelerate the improvement of eye troubles.

The Macrobiotic Approach to Ear Diseases

The Principal Causes of Deafness

A. Looseness of the Eardrum. In order for a drum to create a clear, sharp sound, its skin must be tight. The same is true of the ear. If the eardrum is loose, it will not conduct sound well. Looseness of the eardrum is caused by the overconsumption of liquid and other yin foods. If you feel wetness when you insert a finger into your ear, your hearing may be from ten to thirty percent below normal.

B. Clogged Auditory Ossicles. The *auditory ossicles* are three small bones located in the middle ear which amplify and transmit sound vibrations. These tiny bones are named for their shape, and are called the *hammer, anvil,* and *stirrup.* If they become clogged with sticky fat or mucus, their vibrating ability will be impaired and sound will not be transmitted well. This blockage is usually caused by the overconsumption of mucus- or fat-forming foods such as animal fat, dairy products, sugar, fruits and fruit juice, and nuts and nut butters.

C. Problems with the Cochlea. The cochlea is a tiny, spiral-shaped, bony organ deep within the inner ear containing a fluid which transmits sound vibrations. If the quantity of this liquid changes, or if it becomes thick and sticky, the transmission of sound will be impaired. The foods which cause this problem are often the same as those which produce trouble in the ossicles, particularly extremely yin foods which have the effect of thickening or "freezing" this internal liquid. Sugar, cold iced drinks, Vitamin C, and drugs and medications can have this effect.

D. Auditory Nerve Damage. This nerve, resembling a fine hair, vibrates in response to sound impulses, and then transmits these impulses to the auditory centers of the brain. If it is coated with fat or mucus or if it is swollen, it loses its sensitivity to these sound vibrations. In this case the nerve is not vibrated by incoming sound and thus the impulses are not transmitted to the brain. This condition results from the overconsumption of yin foods, and is similar to the above problems.

In most cases, deafness results from clogged auditory ossicles. An operation to remove mucus and fat deposits is the present medical approach to this problem, but, without a change in diet, the condition often returns. The worst food for our hearing and ear condition is ice cream, which is presently the number one dessert in America, even during the cold winter months. You may notice that your ears ring even after eating several spoonfuls.

A clogged or sticky inner ear condition can be relieved by eliminating foods which produce mucus or fat, such as dairy, sugar, saturated animal fat, fruit juice, and by observing the standard macrobiotic way of eating. Within the standard way of eating, the intake of liquid should be moderate. Along with proper diet, repeated ginger compresses around the ears will help to melt these deposits. Wax deposits stuck inside the ear can be removed by the application of several drops of warm sesame oil from an eyedropper, followed by a warm *bancha* tea rinse, in which a pinch of sea salt has been added. Banging the sides of the head above the ears is also helpful, and you can directly stimulate the ears by covering them with the palm of one hand and tapping hard with two fingers of the other. Do this between fifty and one hundred times. These simple exercises are often included in the practice of *Dō-In*, or self-massage. Since the ears correlate with the kidneys, these treatments will benefit their condition as well.

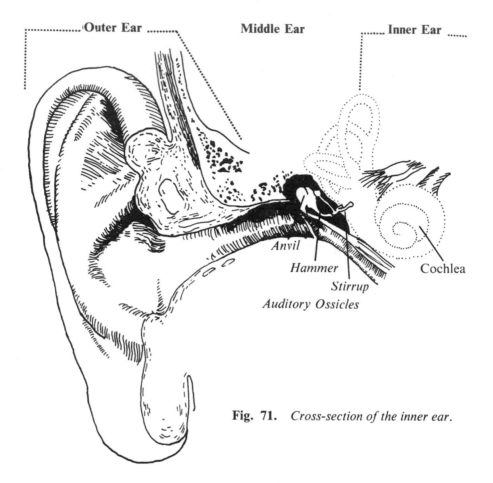

Outer Ear ....   **Middle Ear**   ...... Inner Ear ......

Anvil

Hammer

Stirrup

Cochlea

Auditory Ossicles

Fig. 71. *Cross-section of the inner ear.*

The Teeth

Tooth enamel is harder than bone tissue. The *dentine*, located under the enamel, is similar to bone, but is not composed of bone cells. It is also harder than bone. The central part of the tooth, or *pulp*, contains nerves and blood vessels and is the softest part. Tooth decay can arise when the quality of the saliva or the blood is poor.

Saliva should be slightly alkaline, but if it becomes more yin or acidic, it starts to melt the enamel of the teeth. You can see how this works if you have a tooth that has fallen out. Soak it in a glass of Coca-Cola or any other soft drink overnight. By the following day, the tooth will already have started to soften and decay. If it had been placed in a glass of salt water, however, this would not have happened.

If the quality of the blood is not good, the dentine will start to weaken and will easily chip. Many types of bacteria live in healthy saliva, producing enzymes that are beneficial to the teeth. However, in acidic or unbalanced saliva, a different

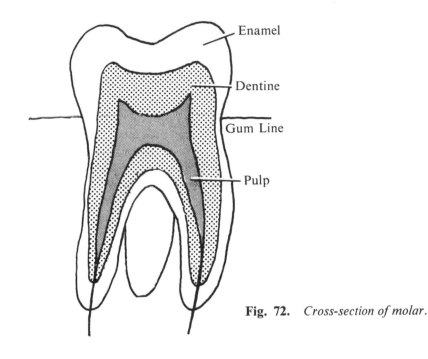

Fig. 72. *Cross-section of molar.*

quality of bacteria flourish which attack and weaken the teeth, resulting in tooth decay. The original cause of both types of tooth decay is an improper quality of blood resulting from the intake of foods like meat, sugar, fruits, drugs, and other acid-forming foods. The best way to care for the teeth is to avoid these items as much as possible and to eat whole grains, beans, cooked vegetables and other macrobiotically-prepared natural foods.

Tooth pain arises when either the nerve or the gum is exposed as a result of decay. Also, when the nerve becomes swollen, it exerts pressure that causes pain. For relief the nerve must be contracted by eating more yang food such as *gomasio* or *umeboshi* plums. Also, eat a little salt every ten to thirty minutes and at the same time apply *dentie* (roasted eggplant and sea salt powder) to the tooth. Within two hours your blood will become yang, causing the nerve to contract and the pain to disappear.

Healthy gums are pink. Red gums are caused by expanded blood capillaries resulting from the intake of expansive foods, including drugs and medications. An opposite condition is *scurvy*, which is caused by an excessive consumption of meat, eggs, and salt without enough yin factors, such as green leafy vegetables, to balance. If we eat a more balanced diet, this condition will not arise. Foods like hard, leafy greens, hard root vegetables, and hard seaweeds are good for strengthening the teeth, particularly the dentine portion.

To clean the teeth, use *dentie*, sea salt, or clean soil. If you binge on sugar, gargle as soon as you can with salted *bancha* tea or salt water, to re-establish the alkaline condition of your saliva. Natural-bristle toothbrushes made from rice or wheat straw, animal hair, or other natural materials are recommended for tooth care.

The structure of the teeth reflects the order of the universe. We have thirty-two teeth which correlate to the thirty-two vertebrae of the spine. Together these equal sixty-four, the number of hexagrams recorded in the *I Ching*, which is an ancient oriental book on practical cosmology. Our permanent teeth show the biological history of man and the types of foods that we are best suited to eat. Of the thirty-two teeth, we have twenty molars which are used primarily for grinding grain, as well as eight incisors which are most effective for cutting vegetables. The four canine teeth can be used for tearing flesh or animal foods. Accordingly, twenty-eight of our teeth, the molars and incisors, are suited for vegetable quality foods, while the four canines can be used for animal foods, in a ratio of seven to one. Five parts of our diet should therefore consist of whole grain cereals, two parts should be vegetables, and one part can include animal food.

Human biological history is the result of eating cereals as main foods, to which supplemental vegetables were added. As shown in the structure of our teeth, animal foods comprised only minor portions of the diet. In fact, they were mainly used only for relatively short periods to balance extremely cold environmental conditions such as those produced by the Ice Ages, and not as long-term principal foods. (See Fig. 73.)

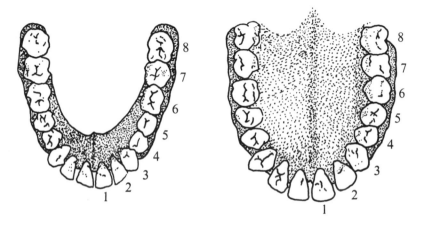

		Age Teeth Appear	Type of Food
1.	Central Incisor	6–8 yrs.	Vegetable
2.	Lateral Incisor	7–9 yrs.	Vegetable
3.	Canine	9–11 yrs.	Animal
4.	1st Pre Molar	9–10 yrs.	Grain and Hard Fiber Food
5	2nd Pre Molar	10–12 yrs.	Grain and Hard Fiber Food
6.	1st Molar	6–7 yrs.	Grain and Hard Fiber Food
7.	2nd Molar	11–13 yrs.	Grain and Hard Fiber Food
8.	3rd Molar (Wisdom Teeth)	17–21 yrs.	Grain and Hard Fiber Food

Fig. 73. *Teeth and corresponding foods.*

If you are eating well, it is often unnecessary to have cavities filled, provided that the condition of your saliva remains slightly alkaline. Tooth decay will be arrested or halted in this type of environment. Avoid having a tooth removed if the roots are still in good condition, since pulled teeth tend to produce an irritable mental or emotional disposition.

Teeth that slant inward show that an abundance of more yang foods were consumed during childhood, while protruding teeth are caused by excessive quantities of yin. If the teeth are chaotic—some slanting inward while others are slanting outward—a person's way of eating was also chaotic, with extremes of both in the diet. Teeth that overlap usually result from the jaw being too contracted. This is caused by too many yang foods. Spaces between teeth are caused by yin. There is an old oriental saying that if you have spaces between the teeth you will not be present at the death of your parents, since these were considered to be signs of separation.

In the chapter, *The Way of Diagnosis*, we studied the pressure point under the middle of the jawbone which can be used to diagnose and treat tooth problems. Strong massage or cigarette moxa on this point will help to relieve any type of tooth disorder. Other helpful treatments include massaging the gums by pressing the outside of the mouth with your fingers, pounding the head, and clicking the teeth. These simple exercises should be repeated about 100 times, and have been used for thousands of years as a part of the practice of *Dō-In*. Gold is the best material for fillings, since it carries a more neutral or balanced charge. Other materials are either slightly more negatively or slightly more positively charged, and therefore tend to alter the normal electromagnetic charge which is generated in the mouth.

The Hair

1. Baldness or Falling Hair

Hair can be compared to a growing plant. If the soil in which plants grow becomes too moist, they can be easily pulled from the ground. The same thing applies to hair. From the sebaceous gland down is the root of the hair. If this region becomes too watery, the hair will begin to fall out. The cause is too much yin in this case, especially liquids and fruit. On the other hand, if good rich soil becomes too dry, like sand, plants can also be easily pulled out. Again, if the root of the hair becomes too dry, it will also fall out. This type of baldness is caused by too much yang in the form of animal food and salt. Baldness, as we can see, can be caused by extremes at either end of the scale.

Drinking excess liquid causes perspiration to form on the forehead because this region correlates with the bladder which discharges liquid. Often, if you continuously drink too much, the hair in the front of the head will start to fall out. This type of baldness is often accompanied by frequent urination. When hair falls out of the center of the head around the hair spiral, the cause is yang—a dry condition resulting from too much animal food and salt. This area of the head correlates to the duodenum and small intestine, and falling hair indicates trouble in these organs. Aside from eating macrobiotically, you can stop balding by applying the juice of *umeboshi* plums to your hair for several days.

2. Grey Hair

Often when a person is anemic, his or her face, nails, and hair start to turn white. This is the result of poor circulation caused by the consumption of too much fat,

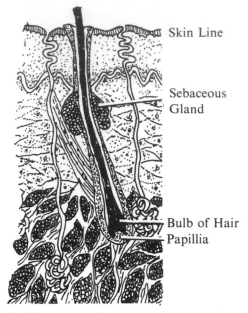

Skin Line

Sebaceous
Gland

Bulb of Hair
Papillia

Fig. 74. *Cross-section of human hair.*

which clogs the arteries and veins, or too much salt which produces constriction. When a person consumes too many animal products like meat, cheese, and eggs, as well as too much salt, the hair will often begin to turn grey or white.

3. Frizzy Hair

This condition is caused by too much yin such as sugar, fruits, fruit juices, and drugs and medications, and indicates that the sexual organs are not functioning well. It can be relieved through the standard macrobiotic way of eating.

4. Split Ends

Splitting hair is also caused by the overconsumption of yin. As in the case of frizzy hair, it indicates that the ovaries or testes have become weak. Since the hair also correlates to the intestinal villi, persons with either condition often suffer from chronic digestive disorders. The standard macrobiotic way of eating will gradually reduce this condition.

5. Dryness

Dry hair is usually caused by too many yang foods, as well as not enough oil. Within the standard way of eating, seaweeds like *kombu*, *hijiki*, and *wakame* are especially good for this condition, particularly when they are cooked for a long period over a low flame. Cook the seaweed with a little oil and *tamari* soy sauce for about four or five hours. This type of preparation will make the seaweed soft, salty, and slightly oily. A small portion eaten daily will produce strong and healthy hair and will normalize the condition of the scalp.

6. Dandruff

Dandruff is nothing but the discharge of excess through the scalp, particularly protein and animal fat. Aside from animal products, overeating in general can produce dandruff. To relieve this condition, begin the standard macrobiotic way of eating, control your intake of food, and chew very well. Your dandruff will soon disappear.

CHAPTER ELEVEN

Natural Pregnancy, Childbirth, and Childcare

Pregnancy

When a woman becomes pregnant, she normally experiences the following physiological, emotional, and psychological changes: (1) Menstruation stops. (2) The breasts and nipples become slightly larger and harder, and are painful when touched. (3) Her taste for food alters. In some cases the desire for items such as brown rice and *miso* diminishes, while the hunger for fruits, sour foods, dairy products, fish, and other items increases. When this occurs, it is best for a woman to follow her intuition while trying to maintain the standard macrobiotoic way of eating. (4) Irritability. (5) Dreams that relate to pregnancy. (6) Morning sickness. This happens when a woman has an overly yin condition. Vomiting is a way of discharging this excess, and to obtain relief, a pinch of *gomasio* or an *umeboshi* plum should be eaten.

The Stages of Pregnancy

A. The Period of the Ovum.   This pre-embryonic period begins with fertilization and continues until the fertilized ovum is implanted in the uterus. It lasts between 8 and 10 days.

B. The Period of the Embryo.   Extending from implantation until the end of the second month, or about 48–50 days from the date of conception, this is the time during which the rudiments of all the organ systems develop, representing a long epoch in the history of the evolution of biological life. A tail emerges during this period, becomes prominent at about the sixth week, and then begins to disappear.

C. The Period of the Fetus.   The following changes occur during this period, which extends from the beginning of the third month through delivery:
   1. Third Month.   The external genitalia differentiate and the sex of the fetus can be determined.
   2. Fourth Month.   Peripheral development occurs at this stage. Hair grows on the head and body, nails appear, and sense organs like the eyes, ears, mouth, and nose develop.
   3. Fifth Month.   Deep internal development occurs during this period, including the formation of blood cells, the development of the bone marrow, and central regions of the internal organs.
   4. Sixth and Seventh Months.   During this stage, the body becomes better proportioned.
   5. Eighth Month.   The fetus continues to grow and to complete its development during this period.
   At full term, the average weight of the embryo is approximately seven pounds.

This represents about a three-billion-times increase in the weight of the original fertilized ovum.

Embryonic Education (Tai-Kyo) (胎教)

In the Orient, the education that a fetus received in the womb was considered far more important than that received after birth. This training was known as *Tai-Kyo*, which means "education during the embryonic period." The following aspects were emphasized as a part of this education.

1. Food

The fertilized ovum increases approximately three billion times in size, or roughly ten million times each day of the nine months of pregnancy. During this time, the quality of its nourishment is entirely dependent on the quality of the mother's blood. Embryological development parallels the evolution of life on earth. It is now estimated that life originally appeared on earth about 3.2 billion years ago. Roughly 2.8 billion years of the evolutionary process were spent in water, while approximately 0.4 billion years of development occurred on land. This 2.8 billion year period corresponds to the 280 days of pregnancy, and the embryo passes through the equivalent of about 10 million years of evolutionary development each day. The process of embryological development generally occurs according to the following logarithmic stages:

1. 7 days—implantation
2. 21 days—formation of major bodily systems
3. 63 days—system development; gland and organ formation
4. 189 days—overall strengthening and development
   280 days total

Because it is developing so rapidly, the fetus is highly susceptible to poisons in its body and its environment. Adults experience a much slower rate of change and can therefore sustain a greater degree of contamination. It is for this reason that, during pregnancy, a mother's eating is of the utmost importance, and she should be especially careful during the first three months (7 days+21 days+63 days). She should satisfy cravings for any particular foods during this time, while trying to maintain the standard macrobiotic way of eating. As much as possible, she should allow her intuition to guide her in the selection of food.

If a pregnant woman takes some type of medication, such as aspirin, sleeping pills, or tranquilizers, or eats an extreme food such as sugar, the effects will probably remain in her body for about three or four days. In this case, however, the embryo must pass through 30 to 40 million years of evolutionary development in a highly chemicalized or polluted environment. In some instances, this may result in congenital deformities such as the absence of limbs or mental retardation.

After the first three months, the baby's constitution has been largely formed. Extreme foods eaten after this tend to affect the more peripheral regions of the body. For example, between the third and fifth months of pregnancy the webbing disappears between the fingers. If a mother eats plenty of yin food during this time, the force of contraction which causes the webbing to disappear is diminished. This can result in a baby being born with webbed fingers.

2. Physical Activity

If a pregnant woman is lazy, her child will often have a similar tendency, while if she keeps busy, her child will develop more active tendencies. Good physical activity will produce a stronger, more compact and active baby.

3. Mental and Spiritual Attitude

If a woman maintains a quiet, peaceful mentality during pregnancy, her child will tend to develop a more gentle personality. However, if she quarrels or frequently becomes angry, her child will have the tendency to become unhappy and experience many difficulties throughout life. The cultivation of a peaceful and happy attitude during pregnancy is as much the responsibility of the father as it is of the mother, since the husband exerts a strong influence on his wife's thoughts and emotions. If a pregnant woman becomes upset, worries, or considers an abortion, the baby will be adversely affected.

Many of us are aware of how thoughts and emotions influence plants. It has been shown that negative thoughts or emotional states adversely affect a plant, while more positive thoughts produce beneficial effects. How much more profound are the mother's thoughts and emotions in their effect on the embryo growing in her body? Thoughts manifest as vibrational wavelengths around the brain, and are particularly active around the midbrain. From there they are transferred along the primary channel (please refer to the section in this book on meridian diagnosis), passing through the *hara* region, which is the area deep within the uterus where implantation occurs. If the mother's thoughts are calm and tranquil, the vibrational environment of the uterus will reflect this harmony. If her thoughts are chaotic and disorderly, however, the embryo will experience this type of vibrational environment. For example, if a mother considers an abortion, the vibrational quality of the uterus will immediately become chaotic, and the fetus will begin to sense possible danger.

In many oriental countries, a newly pregnant woman would begin to make order in her daily life by regularly cleaning her house, washing her clothes, and by preparing herself for the new baby. As much as possible, she tried to avoid books or entertainment that dealt with crime, war, mystery, sex, or other overstimulating subjects. To cultivate her spirituality, she was encouraged to pray and offer her gratitude to her ancestors, nature, and the universe. This sense of order, gratitude and tranquility was transferred to the baby.

Disorders Which May Arise During Pregnancy

1. Bleeding

An excessive intake of either extremely yin or yang foods can cause bleeding. Foods such as salt and animal products may cause the blood to thicken and be discharged, while items such as fruit, liquid, sugar, and spices often cause the capillaries in the ovaries and uterus to weaken and rupture. If the bleeding is caused by excessive yang, begin the standard macrobiotic way of eating, while avoiding animal foods and using a moderate or small amount of salt. For bleeding which results from the opposite cause, begin the standard way of eating, and avoid salads, fruit, and excessive liquid until the condition improves.

2. Miscarriage

A miscarriage can easily occur as a result of the repeated overconsumption of yin foods. When a miscarriage arises very early during pregnancy, it is often mistaken for irregular menstruation. After several years of good eating, a woman can induce a miscarriage during the first several months of pregnancy simply by eating a few pieces of fruit, especially tropical fruits such as figs, avocados, papayas, mangos, and others, along with several glasses of water. These very expansive items will cause the capillaries in the uterus to literally "explode," and the embryo will begin to separate and be discharged. Nosebleeding also results from a similar mechanism. To prevent miscarriage, avoid extremely yin foods during pregnancy. If a miscarriage begins, *miso* soup with *mochi* and scallions should be eaten for several days to help stop it.

3. Premature Birth

Premature birth can be caused by an overly yin condition, as in miscarriage, or by an overly yang condition, during the sixth to eighth months of pregnancy. This often arises as a result of travelling, which is very yangizing. If a woman is eating a balanced diet and maintaining an orderly and peaceful life, this problem should not arise. Ideally, a couple should not have intercourse during pregnancy. However, abstinence is usually difficult. A woman can safely have intercourse up to the end of the sixth month, after which there is a danger of inducing a premature birth.

Childbirth

About 280 days after the onset of the last menstrual period, the fetus is ready for birth into the air world. *Parturition* or *labor* is the process by which the fetus is separated from its mother. It lasts from the time the first contractions begin until the placenta is discharged following the birth of the baby. For women who are pregnant with their first child, labor averages about 16–17 hours among whites, and about 17–18 hours among Negroes. Among *multiparous* women (those who have previously borne one or more children), these figures are respectively about 11 and 12½ hours. With each child, the period of labor tends to shorten. A shorter period of labor indicates that a woman is more yang. Among macrobiotic women, regardless of race, the average is between 8 and 10 hours for the first child and between 4 and 8 hours for the following children.

1. The Stages of Labor

The process of childbirth takes place in the following stages:

A. The First Stage of Labor. Repeated contractions of the uterus force the sac in which the baby is floating, known as the *amniotic sac*, into the cervix. As a result, the cervix dilates, allowing the baby's head to enter the cervical canal. When contractions start to occur at five minute intervals, the sac usually ruptures and the amniotic fluid moistens and lubricates the birth canal. This period, from the first contraction to the breaking of the sac, takes about six hours. This stage corresponds to the time on the earth when biological life shifted from evolutionary development in water to development on land. The period of land formation, during which many earthquakes took place, is replicated in the contractions of the uterus, after which we begin life as a land animal.

B. The Second Stage of Labor. Beginning with the complete dilation of the cervix, this period continues until the baby is separated from its mother. This usually takes up to four hours for most women, while two hours is the average for macrobiotic women.

C. The Third Stage of Labor. After delivery, contractions of the uterus resume, and the placenta separates from the uterine wall and is discharged from the mother's body. This should occur within one-half hour after delivery, and preferably within 15 to 20 minutes. However, if a woman's condition is not strong, this process may take up to six hours. After the placenta is discharged, the uterus continues to contract, causing the ends of the ruptured blood vessels to close.

2. Difficulties with Childbirth and Related Considerations

A. Labor Pains. Pain occurs during delivery when nerves and tissues become expanded from the overconsumption of liquid, sugar, drugs, medications, and other similar items. When contractions begin, these swollen tissues press on the nerves and produce pain. If a woman is in a normal, healthy condition the experience of childbirth should not be painful. Childbirth is normally a very happy event during which a woman should not experience pain.

B. Breech Birth. The baby's head is the most yang part of its body and should emerge from the cervix first. Breech birth means that the feet come out first, and indicates that the head is not compacted or heavy enough to assume a downward position. This results from the mother's overconsumption of expansive foods. If a woman is in good condition, and if the baby is not too large, a breech birth can be performed naturally, without any medication or surgical procedure.

C. Natural Procedures Following Delivery. After birth, infants yangize themselves in adaptation to the air environment which is more expanded that the water environment of the womb. This is partially accomplished by the contractions experienced while passing through the birth canal, and is further completed by the discharge of various excessive factors through crying, which is essential for the baby's survival. If a newborn does not cry immediately, it must be shaken or spanked until crying begins. A baby's first breath is an outbreath, which further contributes toward the process of yangization.

Traditionally, the umbilical cord was cut with bamboo rather than metallic scissors, and was tied with a cotton thread. After the placenta has been discharged, and the mother and baby have been cleaned (the baby should be cleaned with mild warm water), the baby can be held to the mother's breast to begin feeding. For the first several days, the mammary glands secrete a clear fluid known as *colostrum*. Colostrum is not sweet or fatty, and is more yang than milk. It serves to further yangize the baby and provides a natural resistance to a variety of diseases. The baby will often decrease slightly in weight during the first several days, and upon completion of this stage of adaptation, it begins to receive sweet milk.

After delivery, women traditionally drank *tamari-bancha* or thick *miso* soup with *mochi* in order to speed the natural process of recovery and to aid in the adequate production of breast milk.

D. Participation of the Father. In traditional cultures, it was felt that childbirth was something that a husband or father should not directly participate in. Childbirth was considered to be a private matter, and something that ideally should be shared among women. Traditionally, men were usually not present in the delivery room, and the baby was delivered with the assistance of an experienced midwife. Traditional people felt that a husband's attraction for his wife could diminish as a result of his direct participation in the birth experience.

E. Hospital Birth. If you decide to have your baby in a hospital, it is usually necessary to clarify several points beforehand with your doctor or the hospital staff, in order to insure that the birth will be as natural and uncomplicated as possible.
1. Medication should be avoided unless absolutely necessary, including any type of anesthesia, silver nitrate—which is normally put in the baby's eyes to prevent infection as a result of venereal disease—or vitamin supplements.
2. The baby should not be fed artificial formula or glocose solution but should be brought to the mother as soon as possible for breast-feeding. This is therapeutic for the mother as it helps the uterus contract to its normal size. It is advisable to state clearly that you do not wish to receive the medication that is usually given to terminate the production of breast milk.
3. State clearly whether or not you want the baby to be circumcised.

F. Twins. Twins can be either *diovular* or *monovular*. Diovular twins, also known as "false" twins, result from the separate fertilization of two ova by two sperm. This type of fertilization indicates that a woman has a generally more yin condition, and about 75% of all twins belong to this type. Monovular or "identical" twins develop from a single fertilized ovum which splits into two. This can occur in one of two ways: (1) A more yang way, in which the fertilized ovum contains two nuclei. This is similar to chicken eggs which contain two yolks. (2) A more yin way in which two separate masses develop as the fertilized ovum moves through the Fallopian tubes.

Diovular, or *fraternal*, twins are usually very different from each other, but monovular twins are considered to be identical. If you observe them closely, however, you will notice that one is more active or yang, while the other is usually more quiet or yin. Identical twins serve to balance each other during the equivalent of the roughly three billion years of biological evolution that they spend together in the womb. After birth, they usually continue to be attracted to each other through strong psychological and spiritual bonds, similar in many ways to the attraction between husband and wife. Identical twins often have unusual experiences with each other throughout life. For example, if one becomes sick, the other often senses that something is wrong.

Multiple births are not normal for human beings. In some traditional societies, it was even considered unhealthy for a woman to bear twins. A woman who gives birth to twins may often produce more than one set during her life. The tendency to have twins usually skips a generation. This is also often true in cases of so-called "hereditary" diseases and arises because of the tendency of yin to produce yang and vice versa. For example, suppose one generation eats more yang types of food and as a result gives birth to more yang children. These in turn will be attracted to more yin mates as well as more yin food, and they will consequently give birth to a third generation of children having more yin constitutions. These children will in turn be attracted to more yang types of foods, as were their grandparents. It is for this reason that our character and constitution tend to resemble those of our grandparents.

The Newborn Baby

1. Lactation

Breast feeding has many advantages over other types of nourishment, for both infant and mother. Mothers' milk is superior to cows' milk for humans in a variety of ways:

1. It contains a smaller percentage of minerals than does cows' milk. This is the reason that people who drink cows' milk tend to develop a heavier bone structure and grow quickly.
2. It contains less protein than cows' milk, but this protein exists primarily in the form of soluble *lactalbumin*, which is relatively easy to digest. Since the *caseinogen* contained in cows' milk is relatively insoluble in the human digestive system, it often coagulates in the stomach and leads to diarrhea and other digestive disorders.
3. The fat contained in mothers' milk is easier for humans to digest and contains less fatty acid than cows' milk.
4. With human milk, the alkaline condition of the body can be maintained without the action of buffers. The repeated intake of cows' milk, which is more acidic, requires the mobilization of minerals leeched from the bones and teeth to serve as buffers in maintaining an alkaline blood condition.
5. The composition of human milk varies during the first several weeks in order to meet the changing needs of the infant.

A Nutritional Comparison between Human Milk and Cows' Milk

Substance	Human Milk	Cows' Milk
	(Percent)	
Water	88.3	87.3
Inorganic Salts	0.2	0.7
Protein	1.5	3.8
Fat	4.0	4.0
Sugars (carbohydrates)	6.0	4.5
Reaction	Alkaline	Acid

In order to secure health and maximum development, the ratio of protein to carbohydrate in our diet should be approximately one to seven. In normal cases, fat is eventually used by the body for energy, as is carbohydrate, and in this analysis, it is added to the percentage of carbohydrate. In human milk, this ratio can be seen as follows:

$$\frac{\text{protein}}{\text{fat}+\text{carbohydrate}} = \frac{1.5}{4.0+6.0} = \frac{1.5}{10.0} = \frac{1}{7}$$

In cows' milk, we observe the following ratio:

$$\frac{\text{protein}}{\text{fat}+\text{carbohydrate}} = \frac{3.8}{4.0+4.5} = \frac{3.8}{8.5} = \frac{2}{5}$$

As seen in Fig. 75, the proportions of the human body reflect the same one-to-seven ratio that exists in human milk, while the body of a cow reflects the two-to-five ratio found in cows' milk. Since our physical development is guided by food, a baby nourished on cows' milk tends to develop a large bone and body structure, similar to that of a cow, while mental development, which is also determined by food, tends to become dull and lacking in sensitivity. Goats' milk is also an inadequate substitute for human milk. Human milk substitutes should be used only if the mother is very sick or in extreme cases where an infant's survival is threatened.

Breast feeding creates a strong psychological and emotional bond between mother and child, through which both experience a natural feeling of oneness which continues throughout life. Breast-fed children very naturally develop a feeling of love and respect for their mothers, and mothers who breastfeed their children establish a lifelong bond with them.

2. Infant Care

When selecting clothing for a newborn, try to choose all cotton items. Underwear should especially be made of cotton and should be undyed. Try not to overdress your baby. Frequent baths in warm water accelerate a baby's metabolism, and after several weeks a baby can be taken outdoors. Never place an infant in direct sunlight,

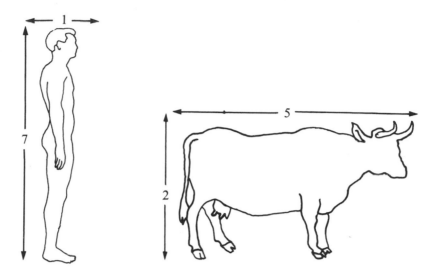

Fig. 75. *The human body generally reflects the one-to-seven ratio found also in human milk, while the form of a cow reflects the two-to-five ratio found in cow's milk.*

since this is too yang for a newborn.

A baby will cry when it is hungry, when it is discharging urine or when it is having a bowel movement. Soiled diapers should be changed immediately, otherwise the child will become accustomed to discomfort and can easily develop a disorderly personality. A baby should sleep on its back. A face-down position is normal for young animals, but not for humans. The normal sleeping position for an adult is either on the back or the side.

Difficulties experienced by a nursing infant are the direct result of the mothers' eating and way of life. If, for example, a nursing infant has diarrhea, the mother has probably been consuming too many yin foods. To correct this, she should eat in a more balanced manner and reduce her liquid intake. Palm-healing can also be helpful, and is done simply by placing one hand over the baby's intestines for several minutes. If a baby has congested lungs and coughs frequently, the mother should drink lotus root tea, while if the baby's urine has an ammonia smell, the mother is eating too much animal food or seaweed. An infant's bowel movement should be yellow and softer than that of an adult. It should not be sticky. If it is darker, the mother is eating too much salt, while a greenish color indicates an overly-yin condition. In this case, the mother should eat a little more salt.

3.   Difficulties with Breastfeeding

Breast tumors, cysts, cancers, or similar disorders can all be treated in the same general manner. Breast cancer is one of the easiest types of cancers to overcome through proper eating and way of life. Uterine and skin cancer, as well as breast cysts or tumors also respond quickly to changes in diet and way of life. Operations or radiation treatments are not necessary for these conditions.

The dietary approach to these disorders is discussed in the chapter, *The Progres-*

sive Development of Sickness, as are various external applications. A ginger compress should be applied for five minutes only, and immediately followed by a taro potato plaster.

If, during this procedure, a woman experiences pain, the taro plaster should be discontinued and a *tofu* plaster should be used in its place. The taro application can be resumed when the pain subsides. These applications will often cause a cyst or tumor to eventually break through the surface of the skin. Pure sesame oil can be applied to the opening in this case, and the entire area can be covered with a bandage. If this occurs while a woman is breastfeeding, the continued nursing with the affected breast will help to accelerate the healing process.

Women who breastfeed are less likely to develop breast tumors or cancer than women who do not. The modern practice of administering a drug to halt the production of breast milk following delivery may actually serve to increase the likelihood of one of these conditions developing.

Food and the Stages of Human Development

Let us consider the following developmental stages which occur after birth:

1. The Period of the Newborn. This is also known as the *neonatal period*, and extends from birth to about the end of the first month. During this period the infant adapts to his new environment, and growth is guided by mechanical consciousness.

2. Infancy. Sensory awareness develops during this stage, which extends from the first month until the infant stands up (around the 16th month).

3. Childhood. Lasting until puberty, this period can be divided into the following stages: (1) From the age of 1 to 6, known as early childhood or the *milk-tooth* period. (2) From 6 to 10, known as middle childhood or the *permanent-tooth* period. (3) From 10 to puberty, known as late childhood or the *prepubertal* period. During this stage, sentimental or emotional consciousness awakens and starts to unfold.

4. Puberty. Puberty begins for girls with the onset of menstruation around the age of 14 (7×2), while boys attain puberty around the age of 16 (8×2). This reflects the cyclical changes which occur every seven years for women and every eight years for men. The sexual organs become functional during this time and secondary sexual characteristics begin to develop.

5. Adolescence. The period of adolescence extends from puberty until the age of 24 for men (8×3) and until 21 (7×3) for women. During this stage, intellectual consciousness develops.

6. Maturity. Early maturity extends until about age 35. During this time, social consciousness develops and matures. Later maturity lasts until 56 (8×7) for men, and 49 (7×7) for women. It is during this time that our understanding of life and the universe naturally develops.

7. The Terminal Age. Lasting until the age of 125 or longer, it is during this time that we achieve our potential as human beings through the development of supreme or universal consciousness.

The time that we spend in the womb is a biological replica of the evolutionary period during which life developed on earth from a single cell to the first land animals. This period of evolution occurred in a watery environment. Infancy corresponds to the evolutionary development of biological life on land, culminating in the appearance of *homo sapiens*.

During the stages of childhood and puberty, we achieve physical maturity, and following this, development occurs more in the areas of mind and consciousness. During the first two stages, we normally depend for our nourishment on the quality of our mother's milk. During childhood, we begin eating prepared foods, and are no longer directly affected by our mother's condition, although we are dependent on the type of foods that she selects and prepares. We assume the responsibility for selecting and preparing our own food at the time of maturity.

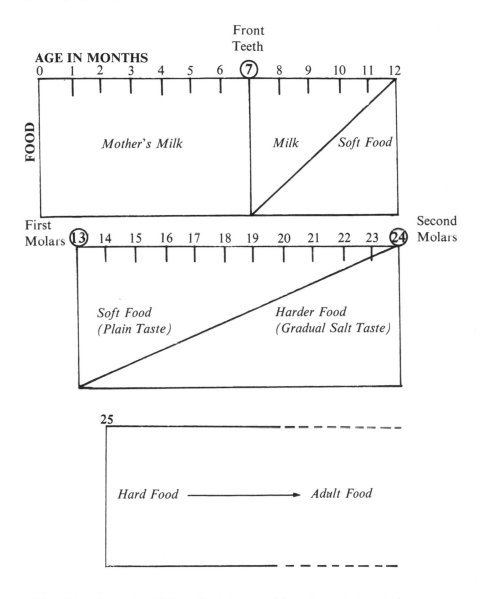

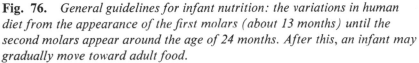

Fig. 76. *General guidelines for infant nutrition: the variations in human diet from the appearance of the first molars (about 13 months) until the second molars appear around the age of 24 months. After this, an infant may gradually move toward adult food.*

Our diet should change in accordance with the development of our teeth. The front teeth appear at about the age of 7–9 months, while the first molars develop around the age of 12–14 months. At about the age of 16–17 months, the canine teeth appear, and the second molars develop at about the age of 20–24 months.

The quantity of breast milk should gradually be decreased at about the age of six months, while the percentage of soft foods, which should contain practically no salt, should gradually be increased. Milk should be stopped around the time the first molars appear (12–14 months). If the child is weaned too soon, he will become stubborn, and if too late, he will become timid and overly-attached to the mother.

The soft foods which the baby should receive include a grain and bean mixture known as *kokkoh*, as well as: (1) soft-cooked rice, prechewed rice, *mochi*, millet, mashed noodles, and oatmeal; (2) vegetables that are either boiled, steamed, or sautéed, and then mashed; (3) mashed beans; (4) mashed seaweed, which may comprise between 5% and 10% of the diet. *Kokkoh* is made from (1) 50% brown rice, (2) 30% sweet brown rice, (3) 15% *azuki* beans, and (4) 5% sesame seeds. To prepare *kokkoh*, roast each of the ingredients separately without burning, add 3 to 4 parts water plus a tiny amount of salt, and cook. Then, mash this mixture in a *suribachi* or a food mill. *Kokkoh* should be more watery for younger babies, and can be used as a substitute for breast milk in emergencies. Infants should receive only a tiny amount of salt or none at all.

Harder foods should be introduced around the time the first molars appear, and by the age of 20–24 months, should comprise the mainstay of the diet. At about the beginning of the third year, a child should receive 1/3 to 1/4 of the amount of salt used by an adult. A child's intake of salt should continue to be less than an adult's until about the 7th or 8th year. (See Fig. 76.)

The Macrobiotic Approach to Children's Diseases

1. Bowed Legs and Knock Knees

Bowed legs result from an overly-expanded condition, and are often the result of feeding. A baby with this condition should be taken outdoors often and should be given less food. Knock knees result from an overly-yang condition, and can be alleviated by making the child's food a little more yin. If a baby has already started to walk and then returns to crawling, this is usually the result of too much salt. It can be relieved by eliminating salt and by making the diet a little more yin.

2. Measles

Every child should have the measles, and the earlier the better. Measles allows a child to discharge the excessive yang that has accumulated during the embryonic period, and if a child does not develop this sickness, his growth will be hindered. After having the measles, a child becomes more yin and begins to grow rapidly.

Measles begins with the appearance of a fever, accompanied by a slight loss of appetite and a feeling of fatigue. The fever usually continues for two or three days, during which time parents often start to worry. Children between the ages of one and two usually have a low fever, but it may be high if the child is older.

Spots usually start to appear within three to four days after the fever begins, but may take up to ten days to appear. Once you know that the child has measles, don't apply any medication or application normally used to reduce fever. Rather than suppressing the fever, we should encourage the discharge of excessive yang by making the surroundings more yin. This can be accomplished by (1) placing a kettle or several steaming pots in the child's room; (2) making the child's room darker; and (3) keeping the windows closed and avoiding exposure to bright sunlight. Cold temperature and bright sunlight can have the effect of suppressing the discharge, and this can be detrimental to the internal organs. If the fever becomes too high (over 103 degrees), place a *tofu* or chlorophyll plaster on the forehead only, and remove it as soon as the fever starts to drop.

If the measles start to disappear after only several days, give the child *daikon* radish drink, which can be made by combining a teaspoon of grated *daikon* with a drop of freshly grated ginger juice and several drops of rice honey or barley malt. Mix in hot water and serve a half teacup. The child can have this drink three or four times a day. These proportions are for a one-year-old child. For a two-year-old, double the quantity of all the ingredients, and for a five-year-old, again double the quantity. This will help to reactivate the discharge.

If the child is coughing excessively, you may prepare brown rice soup with lotus root and the finely chopped skin of a tangerine or mandarin orange. In the beginning stages, the measles appear as red dots which later start to fade into the surrounding skin. If the child's skin becomes itchy during this time, apply pure sesame oil or *daikon* juice for relief.

Mumps

Caused by the consumption of too many yin foods, this is not a necessary disease. It often arises after a child eats several apples, tomatoes, birthday cake, ice cream, or potatoes. The symptoms of mumps include fever and pain behind and underneath the ears, followed several days later by swelling.

For relief, we should try to make the quality of the child's blood more yang. Foods such as burdock, *ume-shoyu-kuzu*, and *gomasio* are helpful for this, as is restricting the intake of liquid. Naturally, all extreme foods should be avoided, and the child should generally stay within the standard macrobiotic way of eating. Be careful, however, not to give the child too much salt.

If the child experiences constipation or blockage in the intestines, an enema made by adding salt to warm water or *bancha* tea can be very helpful. The solution should be less salty than sea water. External applications such as *tofu* or taro plaster can also be applied over the swelling to bring about relief.

Natural Applications

1. **Buckwheat Plaster:** Will draw retained water and excess fluid from swollen areas of the body. Mix buckwheat flour with enough hot water to form a stiff, hard dough and apply, in a half-inch layer, to the affected area. As it draws excess fluid, the dough becomes soft and watery. Replace with a fresh, stiff dough every 3–4 hours.

2. **Brown Rice Cream:** Used to nourish and energize in case of a weakened condition, or when the digestive ability is impaired. Roast brown rice evenly until all the grains turn a yellowish color. To one part rice, add a small amount of sea salt and 3–6 parts water, and pressure cook for at least two hours. Squeeze out the creamy part of the cooked rice gruel with a sanitized cheesecloth. Eat with a small volume of condiment, such as *umeboshi* plum, *gomasio* (sesame salt), *tekka*, kelp or other seaweed powder.

3. **Carp Plaster:** Reduces high fever, as in the case of pneumonia. Crush and mash a whole, live carp, and mix with a small amount of white wheat flour. Spread this mixture onto an oiled paper and apply to the chest. When treating pneumonia, drink one to two teaspoons of carp blood, and then apply the plaster. Take the body temperature every half hour, and immediately remove the carp plaster when the temperature reaches normal.

4. **Daikon Radish Drink:** *Drink No. 1:* Will reduce a fever by inducing sweating. Mix half a cup of grated fresh *daikon* with one tablespoon of *tamari* soy sauce and one quarter teaspoon grated ginger. Pour hot *bancha* tea over this mixture, stir and drink while hot. *Drink No. 2:* To induce urination. Use a piece of cheesecloth to squeeze the juice from the grated *daikon*. Mix two tablespoons of this juice with six tablespoons of hot water to which a pinch of sea salt has been added. Boil this mixture and drink only once a day. Do not use this concoction more than three consecutive days without proper supervision and never use it without first boiling.

5. **Dentie (Denshi):** Prevents tooth problems, promotes a healthy condition in the mouth and stops bleeding anywhere in the body by contracting expanded blood capillaries. Bake an eggplant, particularly the calix or cap, until black. Crush into a powder and mix with 30% to 50% roasted sea salt. Use daily as a tooth powder or apply to any bleeding area—even inside the nostrils in cases of nosebleed—by inserting wet tissue dipped in *dentie* into the nostril.

6. **Dried Daikon Leaves:** Used to warm the body and to treat various disorders of the skin and female sexual organs. Also helpful in drawing odors and excessive oils from the body. Dry fresh *daikon* leaves in the house, away from direct sunlight, until they turn brown and brittle. (If *daikon* leaves are unavailable, turnip greens can be substituted.) Boil 4–5 bunches of the leaves in 4–5 quarts of water until the water

turns brown. Stir in a handful of sea salt and use in one of the following ways:

1. Dip cotton linen into the hot liquid and wring lightly. Apply to the affected area repeatedly, until the skin becomes completely red.
2. Soak in a hot bath in which this mixture has been added.
3. Women experiencing problems in their sexual organs should sit in the bath described above with the water at waist level, the upper portion of the body covered with a towel. Remain in the water until the whole body becomes warm and sweating begins. This generally takes about ten minutes. Repeat as needed, up to ten days.
4. Strain the liquid and use as a douche to eliminate mucus and fat accumulations in the uterine and vaginal regions. This douche can be used after the hot bath described above or by itself.

7. Ginger Compress (Fomentation): Stimulates blood and body fluid circulation and dissolves stagnation. Place grated fresh ginger in a cheesecloth sack and squeeze the ginger liquid into a pot of hot water kept just below the boiling point. Dip a towel into the ginger water, wring it out tightly and apply, hot, directly to the area to be treated. A second, dry towel can be placed on top to reduce heat loss. Apply a fresh hot towel every 2–3 minutes until the skin becomes red.

8. Ginger Sesame Oil: Activates the functions of the blood capillaries, circulation, and nerve reactions. Also relieves aches and pains. Mix grated fresh ginger with an equal amount of sesame oil. Dip cotton linen into this mixture and rub briskly into the skin of the affected area.

9. Gomasio (Sesame Salt): Strengthens digestion, intestinal absorption and blood quality. Will also relieve general fatigue and such pains as headache and toothache. For medicinal use mix 3–4 parts roasted sesame seeds with one part roasted sea salt. (For daily use as a condiment, use 8–14 parts sesame seeds to one part sea salt.) Grind both in a *suribachi* (mortar and pestle) slowly and evenly, crushing all seeds, but not completely into a powder. Take one teaspoon of *gomashio* once or twice a day for several days. This may be used with hot *bancha* twig tea or with hot water, sprinkled on cereal grains during the meal.

10. Grated Daikon: A digestive aid, especially for fatty, oily, heavy foods, and for animal food. Grate fresh *daikon* (red radish or turnip can be used if *daikon* is not available). Sprinkle with *tamari* soy sauce and eat about a tablespoonful.

11. Scallion, Onion, or Daikon Juice: Will neutralize the poison of a bee sting or an insect bite. Cut either a scallion, onion or *daikon*, or their greens, and squeeze out the juice. (If you cannot obtain these vegetables, red radish can be used.) Rub the juice thoroughly into the wound.

12. Kuzu (Kudzu) Drink: Strengthen digestion, increases vitality and relieves general fatigue. Dissolve a heaping teaspon of *kuzu* powder into one cup of cold water. Bring the mixture to a boil, reduce the heat to the simmering point and stir constantly until the liquid becomes a transparent gelatin. Now stir in one teaspoon of *tamari* soy sauce and drink while hot.

13. Lotus Root Plaster: Draws stagnated mucus from the sinuses, nose, throat and bronchi. Mix grated fresh lotus root with 10%–15% pastry flour and 5% grated fresh ginger. Spread a half-inch layer onto cotton linen and apply the lotus root directly to the skin. Keep on for several hours or overnight, and repeat daily for several days. A ginger compress can be applied before this application to stimulate circulation and to loosen mucus in the area you are treating.

14. Mustard Plaster: Stimulates blood and body fluid circulation and loosens stagnation. Add hot water to dry mustard and stir well. Spread this mixture onto a paper towel, and sandwich it between two thick cotton towels. Apply this "sandwich" until the skin becomes red and warm, and then remove.

15. Ranshio: Used to strengthen the heart, and to stimulate heartbeat and blood circulation. Crush a raw egg and mix with one tablespoon of *tamari* soy sauce. Drink slowly. Use only once a day and for no more than three days.

16. Raw Brown Rice and Seeds: Will eliminate worms of various types. Skip breakfast and lunch. Then, on an empty stomach, eat a handful of raw brown rice with a half-handful of raw seeds such as pumpkin or sunflower seeds, and another half-handful of chopped raw onion, scallion or garlic. Chew everything very well, and have your regular meal later in the day. Repeat for 2 to 3 days.

17. Salt Bancha Tea: Used to loosen stagnation in the nasal cavity or to cleanse the vaginal region. Add enough salt to warm *bancha* tea (body temperature) to make it just a little less salty than sea water. Use the liquid to wash deep inside the nasal cavity through the nostrils, or as a douche. Salt *bancha* tea can also be used as a wash for problems with the eyes.

18. Salt Pack: Used to warm any part of the body. For relief of diarrhea, for example, apply the pack to the abdominal region. Roast salt in a dry pan until hot and then wrap in a thick cotton linen or towel. Apply to the troubled area and change when the pack begins to cool.

19. Salt Water: Cold salt water will contract the skin in the case of burns, while warm salt water can be used to clean the rectum, colon and vagina. When the skin is damaged by fire, immediately soak the burned area in cold salt water until irritation disappears. Then apply vegetable oil to seal the wound from the air. For constipation or mucus and fat accumulations in the rectum, colon, and vaginal regions, use warm salt water (body temperature) as an enema or douche.

20. Sesame Oil: Use to relieve stagnated bowels or to eliminate retained water. Take one to two tablespoons of raw sesame oil on an empty stomach to induce the discharge of stagnated bowels. To eliminate water retention in the eyes, put a drop or two of pure sesame oil in the eyes with an eyedropper, preferably before sleeping. Continue up to a week, until the eyes improve. Before using the sesame oil for this purpose, boil and then strain it with a sanitized cheesecloth to remove impurities.

21.   Tamari Bancha Tea: Neutralizes an acidic blood condition, promotes blood circulation and relieves fatigue. Pour one cup of hot *bancha* twig tea over one to two teaspoons of *tamari* soy sauce. Stir and drink hot.

22.   Taro Potato Plaster (Albi Plaster):   Draws pus and stagnated blood from tumors, boils and similar eruptions. After paring the skin, grate the white interior of the taro potato and mix with 5% grated fresh ginger. Spread this mixture in a half-inch layer on a piece of cotton linen and apply the potato side directly to the tumor or skin. Change every four hours. A ginger compress can be used before and after this application to warm the body and to increase circulation in the affected area.

23.   Tofu Plaster: Is more effective than an ice pack to draw out a fever. Squeeze the water from the *tofu*, mash it and then add 10%–20% pastry flour and 5% grated ginger. Mix the ingredients and apply directly to the skin. Change every two to three hours.

24.   Umeboshi Plum; Baked Umeboshi Plum; Powdered, Baked Umeboshi Plum Pit: Neutralizes an acidic condition and relieves intestinal problems, including those caused by microorganisms. Take two or three *umeboshi* plums with *bancha* twig tea. Or, you may bake the plums or their pits until black. If you are using the pits, powder them and add a tablespoonful to a little hot water or tea.

25.   Ume-Sho-Bancha: Strengthens the blood and the circulation through the regulation of digestion. Pour one cup of *bancha* tea over the meat of one-half to one *umeboshi* plum and one teaspoon of *tamari* soy sauce. Stir and drink hot.

26.   Ume-Sho-Kuzu (Kudzu) Drink: Strengthens digestion, revitalizes energy and regulates the intestinal condition. Prepare the *kuzu* drink according to the instructions in Number 12, and add the meat of one-half to one *umeboshi* plum along with the soy sauce. An eighth of a teaspoon of grated fresh ginger may also be added.

Arthritis

Although its symptoms take various forms, arthritis can be classified into two distinct categories, according to cause:
1. Yin Arthritis—produced by excessive intake of various yin foods such as fruits, fruit juice, especially tropical and semi-tropical varieties, spices, stimulant and aromatic herbs and beverages, soft drinks, sugar, honey, chocolate, and vinegars, as well as excessive intake of tomato, eggplant, and other vegetables of tropical origin.
2. Yang Arthritis—caused by excessive intake of the yang food categories, including meat, eggs, and other animal food. Large amounts of salt and other minerals, including the excessive intake of calcium associated with the regular consumption of dairy foods, also creates a yang arthritic condition.

Despite these differences, however, both types of arthritis are aggravated to varying degrees by the consumption of excessive oil and fat from either animal or vegetable sources. In addition, both types are accelerated by excessive intake of liquid and icy cold drinks such as soda, beer and other cold beverages. Ice cream is of course one of the major factors contributing to the symptoms of arthritis.

Dietary Approach: Avoid extreme categories of both yin and yang foods and, in general, follow the standard macrobiotic diet. All food should be cooked, although a third of your vegetables may be lightly or quickly cooked. The consumption of both animal food and fruit should be minimized. The use of salt, *miso*, *tamari* and other salty seasonings and condiments should be moderate.
1. When selecting vegetables, it is advisable to avoid potatoes, tomatoes, eggplant, asparagus, spinach, avocados, beets, zucchini squash and mushrooms. The main food in the daily diet should be whole grains, while supplemental foods should include cooked vegetables, beans, seaweed, and if desired, small portions of animal food such as fish and seafood, and an occasional small volume of cooked or dried fruits. The proportion of the main or principal food to side dishes should be 2:1.
2. As a special therapeutic dish, cook dried, shredded *daikon* with *miso* or *tamari* soy sauce to taste. *Miso* and scallion cooked together with several drops of sesame oil is also beneficial when used as a frequent condiment.

The use of such wild plants as dandelion and watercress can also be helpful. Prepare them by first sautéing with a small amount of sesame oil, then adding a little water and simmering.
3. Arthritis is commonly accompanied by chronic intestinal disorders. Thorough chewing of food is therefore especially important, preferably 80 to 100 times or more per mouthful, until the food becomes completely liquified.
4. The symptoms of arthritis can be treated by applying a hot ginger compress once each day to joints or hardened body parts in order to accelerate blood and body fluid circulation and to dissolve stagnation. It is also helpful to soak swollen fingers and hands, or feet, in very hot ginger water for about 10 minutes.
5. Another helpful external treatment for arthritic persons is the daily or fre-

quent application of a ginger compress on the abdominal area. A further recommendation is to rub down and along the spine with hot ginger water. Soak a towel in the water, squeeze, and then rub the area until it becomes red. It is also very helpful to mix one teaspoon *umeboshi* plum that has been baked and then crushed into a black powder, with a small cup of *bancha* twig tea. Take daily or once every two or three days depending upon the severity of the symptoms.

It is important to make cereal grains the main food around which the rest of the diet centers. These include rice, millet, barley, rye, wheat and oats, among others. These grains should be eaten primarily in their whole form rather than as a flour.

Principles of the Order of the Universe

The Seven Universal Principles of the Infinite Universe

1. Everything is a differentiation of one Infinity.
2. Everything changes.
3. All antagonisms are complementary.
4. There is nothing identical.
5. What has a front has a back.
6. The bigger the front, the bigger the back.
7. What has a beginning has an end.

The Twelve Laws of Change of the Infinite Universe

1. One Infinity manifests itself into complementary and antagonistic tendencies, yin and yang, in its endless change.
2. Yin and yang are manifested continuously from the eternal movement of one infinite universe.
3. Yin represents centrifugality. Yang represents centripetality. Yin and yang together produce energy and all phenomena.
4. Yin attracts yang. Yang attracts yin.
5. Yin repels yin. Yang repels yang.
6. Yin and yang combined in varying proportions produce different phenomena. The attraction and replusion among phenomena is proportional to the difference of the yin and yang forces.
7. All phenomena are ephemeral, constantly changing their constitution of yin and yang forces; yin changes into yang, yang changes into yin.
8. Nothing is solely yin or solely yang. Everything is composed of both tendencies in varying degrees.
9. There is nothing neuter. Either yin or yang is in excess in every occurrence.
10. Large yin attracts small yin. Large yang attracts small yang.
11. Extreme yin produces yang, and extreme yang produces yin.
12. All physical manifestations are yang at the center, and yin at the surface.

Examples of Yin and Yang

	▽	△
	YIN	*YANG*
Characteristic	*Centrifugal Force*	*Centripetal Force*
Tendency	Expansion	Contraction
Function	Diffusion	Fusion
	Dispersion	Assimilation
	Separation	Gathering
	Decomposition	Organization

[193]

Characteristic	▽ YIN Centrifugal Force	△ YANG Centripetal Force
Movement	More inactive, slow	More active, fast
Vibration	Shorter wave, higher frequency	Longer wave, lower frequency
Direction	Ascent, vertical	Descent, horizontal
Position	More outward and peripheral	More inward and central
Weight	Lighter	Heavier
Temperature	Colder	Hotter
Light	Darker	Brighter
Humidity	More wet	More dry
Density	Thinner	Thicker
Size	Longer	Smaller
Shape	More expansive, fragile	More contractive, harder
Form	Longer	Shorter
Texture	Softer	Harder
Atomoc particle	Electron	Proton
Elements	N, O, K, P, Ca, etc.	H, C, Na, As, Mg, etc.
Environment	Vibration . . . Air . . . Water . . . Earth	
Climatic effects	Tropical climate	Colder climate
Biological	More vegetable quality	More animal quality
Sex	Female	Male
Organ structure	More hollow and expansive	More compacted and condensed
Nerves	More peripheral, orthosympathetic	More central, parasympathetic
Attitude	More gentle, negative	More active, positive
Work	More psychological, and mental	More physical and social
Dimension	Space	Time

Abehsera, Michel. *Cooking for Life*. Binghamton, N. Y.: Swan House.

Aihara, Cornellia. *Chico-San Cookbook*, Chico. Calif.: Chico-San, Inc.

Aihara, Cornellia, *The Dō of Cooking*, 4 vols. Oroville, Calif.: George Ohsawa Macrobiotic Foundation.

Carrel, Alexis. *Man the Unknown*. New York: Harper and Row.

Chishima, Kikuo. *Revolution of Biology and Medicine*. Gifu, Japan: Neo-Haematological Society Press.

Colbin, Annemarie. *The Book of Whole Meals*. Brookline, Mass.: Autumn Press.

Dufty, William. *Sugar Blues*. New York: Warner Publications.

East West Foundation. *A Dietary Approach to Cancer Accorldng to the Principles of Macrobiotics*. Brookline, Mass.: East West Publications.

East West Foundation. *A Nutritional Approach to Cancer*. Ibid.

East West Foundation. *Cancer and Diet*. Ibid.

East West Foundation. *Macrobiotic Case Histories*. Vols. I through VI. Ibid.

East West Foundation. *Report on the First North American Congress of Macrobiotics*. Ibid.

East West Foundation. *Standard Recommendations for Diet and Way of Life*. Ibid.

Esko, Wendy. *Introducing Macrobiotic Cooking*. Tokyo: Japan Publications, Inc.

Fukuoka, Masanobu. *The One-Straw Revolution: An Introduction to Natural Farming*. Emmaus, Pa: Rodale Press.

Gilbert, Margaret Shea. *Biography of the Unborn*. New York: Hafner.

Jacobsen and Brewster. *The Changing American Diet*. Washington, D. C.: Center for Science in the Public Interest.

Kohler, Jean and Mary Alice. *Healing Miracles from Macrobiotics*. West Nyack, N. Y.: Parker Publishing Co.

Kushi, Michio. *Acupuncture: Ancient and Future Worlds*. Brookline, Mass.: East West Foundation.

Kushi, Michio. *Oriental Diagnosis*. London: Sunwheel, Ltd.

Kushi, Michio. *How to See Your Health: The Book of Diagnosis*, Tokyo: Japan Publications, Inc.

Kushi, Michio. *Natural Healing Through Macrobiotics*. Ibid.

Kushi, Michio. *The Teachings of Michio Kushi*, Vols. I and II. Ibid.

Kushi, Michio. *The Book of Macrobiotics: The Universal Way of Health and Happiness*. Tokyo: Japan Publications, Inc.

Kushi, Michio. *The Book of Dō-In: Exercise for Physical and Spiritual Developmen* Ibid.

Kushi, Aveline. *How to Cook with Miso*. Ibid.

Mendelsohn, Robert S., M. D. *Confessions of a Medical Heretic*. Chicago. Ill.: Contemporary Books.

Muramoto, Noboru. *Healing Ourselves*. New York: Avon; London: Michael Dempsey/Cassell.

Ohsawa, George. *Acupuncture and the Philosophy of the Far East*. Boston, Mass.: Tao Books.

Ohsawa, George. *The Book of Judgment*. Los Angeles: Ohsawa Foundation.

Ohsawa, George. *Cancer and the Philosophy of the Far East*. Binghamton, N. Y.: Swan House.

Ohsawa, George. *Guidebook for Living*. Los Angeles: Ohsawa Foundation.

Ohsawa, George. *Practical Guide to Far-Eastern Macrobiotic Medicine*. Oroville, Calif.: George Ohsawa Macrobiotic Foundation.

Ohsawa, George. *The Unique Principle*. Ibid.

Ohsawa, George. *Zen Macrobiotics*. Los Angeles: Ohsawa Foundation.

Ohsawa, Lima. *The Art of Just Cooking*. Tokyo: Autumn Press.

Sacks, Castelli, Donner, and Kass. "Plasma Lipids and Lipoproteins in Vegetarians and Controls." Boston: *New England Journal of Medicine*. May 29, 1975.

Sacks, Rosner, and Kass. "Blood Pressure in Vegetarians." *American Journal of Epidemiology*, Vol. 100, No. 5, Baltimore: Johns Hopkins University.

Sakurazawa, Nyoiti (George Ohsawa), edited by Dufty, William. *Macrobiotics*. London: Tandem Books. Published in the U.S.A. under the title *You Are All Sanpaku*. New York: University Books.

Select Committee on Nutrition and Human Needs, U.S. Senate. *Dietary Goals for the United States*. February 1977.

Stiskin, Nahum. *The Looking Glass God*. Tokyo: Autumn Press.

Surgeon General's Report on Health Promotion and Disease Prevention. *Healthy People*. Washington, D. C. September, 1979.

Veith, Ilza. *The Yellow Emperor's Classic of Internal Medicine*. Berkely, Calif.: University of California Press.

Wilhelm and Baynes. *I Ching*. Princeton: Princeton University Press.

Yamamoto, Shizuko. *Barefoot Shiatsu*. Tokyo: Japan Publications, Inc.

Periodicals

East West Journal. Brookline, Mass.

Kushi Institute Study Guide, Kushi Institute Newsletter, Brookline, Mass.

The Order of the Universe. Brookline, Mass. East West Foundation.

Nutrition Action, Washington D. C.: Center for Science in the Public Interest.

The Macrobiotic Review. Baltimore, Md.: East West Foundation.

Spiral. Community Health Foundation, London.

Le Compas. Paris.

About the Author

Michio Kushi was born in Kokawa, Wakayama-Ken, Japan in 1926. His early years were devoted to the study of international law at Tokyo University, and an active interest in world peace through world federal government in the period following the Second Word War. It was during this time that he encountered Yukikazu Sakurazawa, the well-known teacher of oriental medicine and philosophy, known in the West as George Ohsawa. Inspired by Mr. Ohsawa's teaching, Mr. Kushi began his lifelong study of the application of traditional understanding to solving the problems of the modern world.

Mr. Kushi came to the United States in 1949 to pursue graduate studies at Columbia University, and since that time has lectured on oriental medicine, philosophy, culture, and macrobiotics throughout North America, Europe, South America, and the Far East. Through his continuing lectures, seminars, and consultations, Mr. Kushi has guided thousands of people to restore their physical, psychological, and spiritual quality as the fundamental means of achieving world peace. In his unique comprehension of man and the universe, evolved from a deep understanding of law, philosophy, and medicine, he has applied the traditional wisdom of the Far East and other cultures to the modern predicament of biological and social disorder, formulating a dynamic blueprint for the future of mankind.

Michio Kushi lives in Brookline, Massachusetts, with his wife, Aveline, and children. He is the founder of Erewhon, Inc., the leading distributor of natural and macrobiotic foods in North America, as well as the *East West Journal*, a monthly news magazine with over 100,000 readers.

Mr. Kushi is the founder and president of the East West Foundation, a federally-approved, non-profit educational and cultural institution established in Boston in 1972 to help spread and develop all aspects of the macrobiotic way of life through seminars, publications, research, and other means. Under Mr. Kushi's guidance, the Foundation presents regular seminars and study programs in Boston and throughout the United States, and is currently publishing a series of books and periodicals which deal with various aspects of macrobiotics and oriental medicine.

So as to further the development of a truly human medicine along with medical and scientific research for the future benefit of society at large, the Foundation has sponsored periodic seminars and conferences for members of the medical community and for the general public. These have included the conferences, *A Nutritional Approach to Cancer and Major Illnesses* presented in the Boston area, as well as Mr. Kushi's ongoing international seminars on macrobiotic and oriental medicine. The proceedings of these conferences have been published and distributed to leading medical and scientific institutions throughout the world.

In 1977, Mr. Kushi and associates, including Dr. Robert Mendelsohn, met in Washington with members of the White House domestic policy staff to discuss various proposals for improving the food and nutrition policy of the United States. Subsequent discussions were held with several of the individuals who were involved in the preparation of the Senate Nutrition Committee report, *Dietary Goals for the United States*, including Dr. Mark Hegsted, presently with the U.S. Department of Agriculture, Dr. Philip Lee, of the University of California, and others.

At the same time, Mr. Kushi and associates have begun the preliminary steps toward the formation of an East West Foundation Medical and Scientific Advisory Board. The Board is presently comprised of a group of international physicians and related medical professionals who share the Foundation's interest in synthesizing traditional and modern methods of medical practice and understanding.

So as to further the continuing application of macrobiotic principles to a variety of social problems, Mr. Kushi has made several presentations to the United Nations in New York, including an address on *One Peaceful World through Macrobiotics.*

In 1977, Mr. Kushi and associates established the Michio Kushi Institute in London, for the purpose of providing concentrated study programs in various aspects of macrobiotics, oriental medicine, and natural healing. In the following year, Kushi Institutes were established in Amsterdam and Boston with the similar purpose of providing study programs for the qualification of teachers and health consultants capable of solving various individual and social problems.

In the autumn of 1978, Mr. Kushi and associates organized and presented the *First European Congress of Macrobiotics* in London. Attended by delegates from throughout Western Europe, the congress drafted a series of proposals and recommendations aimed at applying macrobiotic principles to the solution of a wide variety of social problems. The European Congress met again in the autumn of 1979 in Antwerp, Belgium, while in the United States, the *First North American Congress of Macrobiotics* was held in August of that year in Boston. Both the European and North American Congresses are scheduled to meet once every year, along with future regional congresses in South America, and the Far East, followed by a *World Congress of Macrobiotics* during the 1980's.

Mr. Kushi's published works in English include: *The Book of Macrobiotics: The Universal Way of Health and Happiness, The Book of Dō-In: Exercise for Physical and Spiritual Development, How to See Your Health: The Book of Oriental Diagnosis,* and *Natural Healing through Macrobiotics, Cancer and Heart Disease: The Macrobiotic Approach to Degenerative Disorders,* published by Japan Publications, Inc., *Oriental Diagnosis,* published by Sunwheel Ltd. in London, and *Visions of a New World: The Era of Humanity,* published by *East West Journal.* In addition, Mr. Kushi has inspired and encouraged a number of other books including *How to Cook with Miso* by Aveline Kushi, *Barefoot Shiatsu* by Shizuko Yamamoto, *Introducing Macrobiotic Cooking* by Wendy Esko, and *Macrobiotic Cooking for Everyone* by Edward and Wendy Esko, published by Japan Publications, Inc., *Healing Miracles from Macrobiotics* by Jean and Mary Alice Kohler, published by Parker Publishing Company, and *Recalled by Life: The Story of My Recovery from Cancer* by Anthony J. Sattilaro, M.D. and Tom Monte, published by Houghton Mifflin Company.

Index

A

Abdomen, 37, 38, 79, 90, 91
Abortion, 145, 146, 175
Absorption, 85
Acetone, 130
Aches, 25
Acid condition, 100
Acid reaction, 93
Acidosis, 109, 130
Acne, 128
Acrodermatitis enteropathica, 5
Acromegaly, 126
Acupuncture, 12, 70
Addison's disease, 8, 127
Additives, 32
Adenoids, 146
Aihara, Mr. and Mrs. Herman, 12
Adolescence, 182
Adrenal glands, 121, 123, 125, 127, 129
Adrenalin, 123, 125
Agar-agar, 36
Agglutination, 109
Agranulocytes, 105
Albi, see Taro potato
Alcohol, 32
Alkalosis, 109
Allergies, 6, 17, 35, 101
Alveoli, 95, 97
Amniocentesis, 7
Amniotic sac, 177
Amoeba, 91, 105
Analgesics, 6
Ancestors, 52, 54, 55
Androgens, 125
Anemia, 9, 105, 106
Aneurysm, 113
Anger, 88
Antibiotics, 100
Antibodies, 114
Anti-insulin, 123
Anus, 61
Aorta, 113
Appendectomy, 10, 46, 145

Appendicitis, 9, 37, 90
Appendix, 145
Applications, natural, 187
Arteries, 112, 113,
Arteriosclerosis, 5, 112, 113
Artherosclerosis, 113
Arthritis, 191
Ascending colon, 42
Aspirin, 13, 174
Asthma, 5, 72, 97
Astigmatism, 10, 71
Atmospheric conditions, 49
Atresia, 156
Auditory nerve, 167
Auditory ossicles, clogged, 167
Autonomic nervous system, 135, 137

B

B-Vitamins, 65, 94
Baby food, 182–184
Bad breath, 103
Baldness, 171, 172
Bancha twig tea, 30; with salt, 189; with tamari soy sauce, 190
Basal metabolism, 123
Basophils, 104, 105
Baths, 31, 93, 188
Baths, hip, 188
Beans, 30
Bedwetting, 50
Belching, 103
Bilateral masectomy, 6
Bile, 89, 114, 115, 123
Birth, see Childbirth
Birth control pills, 124, 140
Bladder, 61
Blindness, 178
Blood, 25, 103, 104, 108, 109, 110, 111, 117
Blood pressure, 112, 116, 117
"Blood Pressure in Vegetarians," 116, 117
Blood sugar, 123, 129, 132, 133
Blood transfusions, 108, 109
Blood type, 108, 109, 115

Blood vessels, 112, 113
Bloodshot, 63
Body odor, 9, 64
Bo-Shin, 58
Bowed legs, 184
Bowel movement, 61, 79, 91, 181
Brain, 42, 46, 56, 135, 139
Breast feeding, 179–184
Breasts, 37, 46
Breech birth, 177
Bronchi, 59, 72, 95
Bronchitis, 72, 97, 98
Brown rice, 30, 187, 189
Buckwheat, 30, 46, 87
Buckwheat plaster, 46, 187
Buddha, 28
Buffer action, 100, 110, 129
Bun-Shin, 64
Butter, 32

C

Caesarian section, 6
Calcified stones, 63
Calcium, 93, 100
Caloric energy, 75
Cancer, 6, 8, 29, 39, 40; brain, 42; breast, 10, 42, 181; colon, 68; etiology of, 10; kidney, 70; liver, 42, 68, 89; lung, 96; pancreas, 42, 68; prostate, 42; rectum, 41; skin, 10, 35, 40 small intestine, 42, 68; spleen, 42, 68; stomach, 9, 41, 88; terminal, 43; thyroid, 7; transverse colon, 42, dietary approach to, 43; treatment by ginger compress, 45; uterine, 10, 42; yin and yang, 41, 42, 44, 105, 114
Carbohydrates, 38, 85, 123
Carbon dioxide, metabolism of, 129
Carbonic acid, 110

Cardiovascular disease, 6, 38
Carp plaster, 99, 187
Carrel, Dr. Alexis, 18
Cataracts, 163
Cellular oxidation, 123
Cereal grains, 30
Cereal grain tea or coffee, 30
Cervix, 177
Chakras, 143, 145
Chancroid venereal diseases,
    161
Channel, primary or spiritual,
    66, 175
Chanting, 149
Cheese, 32
Chemotherapy, 35, 43
Chest congestion, 36
Chest pain, 98
Chewing, 31, 35, 83, 85
Chi-So, 49
Childbirth, 33, 173, 176
Childcare, 173 ff
Chlorophyll, 106
Cholera, 91
Cholesterol, 38, 111, 112
Cigarette moxa, 75
Circulatory system, 39, 83, 84,
    110, 112
Circumcision, 71
Clothing, 31, 146
Cobalt radiation, 43
Cochlea, 167
Coffee, 32
Colds, 98
Colitis, 92
Color blindness, 166
Colostrum, 178
Coma, 130
Communication, 138
Complementary relationships,
    58–62
Complexion, oily, 39
Condiments, 31
Congenital deformities, 174
Constipation, 91
Consciousness, 55, 138, 182
Constitution, 27, 58
Convulsions, 129
Coronary bypass, 7
Coronary circuit, 110
Corpus luteum, 124, 157
Corsican seaweed, 87
Cortex, 138
Cortisone, 137
Coughing, 34, 98, 100

Cramps, 88, 92, 126
Cranial nerves, 135
Crawling, 184
Cretinism, 126
Crossed eyes, 165
Culture, 139
Cyclical changes, in women
    and men, 182

D

Daikon, 187, 188
Daikon application, 34
Daikon drink, 187
Daikon leaves, 107, 159, 187
Dairy products, 32
Dan-Chu, 71
Dandelion tea, 30
Dandruff, 172
Deafness, 36, 167
Deformities, 174
Degenerative sicknesses, 26
Delivery procedure following,
    178
Dentie, 113, 169
Dentine, 183
Depression, 80
Dermoid cysts, 160
Descending colon, 42
Detachment of retina, 163
Development, human, and
    food, 181–184
Diabetes, 126, 129 130, 131,
    132, 133
Diagnosis, 49–81
Diagnosis points, 71, 72, 74
Diaphragm, 62
Diarrhea, 34, 91
Diastolic pressure, 116
Diet, macrobiotic standard,
    29
Diet, modern, 17, 32
"Dietary Goals for the United
    States," 30
Digestion, 83, 119
Digestive system, 55, 61, 83,
    86
Disaccharides, 93
Discharge, 34
DNA, 55, 141, 143
Do-In, 12, 168, 171
Douche, 159, 188
Drugs, 32, 46
Dualistic monism, 18
Ductus deferens, 153

Dulse, 30
Duodenum, 120, 123, 125,
    129
Dufty, William, 94
Dwarfism, 126
Dysentery, 91, 92

E

E. coli meningitis, 5
Ear, 36, 71, 167
Earth's force, 20, 66, 67,
    120, 143, 145
Eating, 9, 27, 28, 29, 102
Echerichia, 92
Eczema, 5
Education, embryonic, 174
Efferent ducts, 153
Eggplant, 32
Eggs, 32
Egocentricity, 140
Ejaculation, 153
Electromagnetic energy, 65
Electroshock, 7
Eliminatioh, 33
Embryo, 67, 103, 173, 174
Emotions, 25, 34
Emphysema, 95
Endocrine system, 119, 120,
    121, 124, 125, 127, 128
Enema, 185
Energy, 65, 67, 143, 145
Enteritis, 91
Environment, harmony with,
    29
Enzymes, 85
Eosinophils, 104, 105
*Epidemiology, American
    Journal of*, 117
Epididymis, 153, 154
Epinephrine, 123
Epilepsy, 150, 151
Episiotomy, 6
Erythrocytes, 103
Esophagus, 83
Estrogens, 124, 125, 127
Excess, discharge and
    accumulation of, 33, 38
Excretory system, 83
Exercise, 31
Expression, 57, 140
Eyes, 59, 62, 63, 126, 136, 163,
    164, 165

F

Face, 39, 80, 163
Fallopian tubes, 38, 155
Farsightedness, 165
Fasting, 88, 89
Father's influence, 55
Fatigue, 24
Fats, 38, 85, 112, 113
Fatty acids, 39, 94
Female reproductive system,
    155, 158
Fertilization, 156, 173
Fetus, 173
Fever, 34, 184
Finger pressure, 74
Fingernails, 61, 62, 87
Fingers, webbed, 175
Fish, 30
Five transformations, 75
Flour products, 34
flu vaccine, 7
Follicles, 155, 156
Foods, yin and yang, 32
Forebrain, 137
Forgetfulness, 25
Formed elements, 103
Formula feeding, 5, 6
Fruits, 30, 32
Future, 138, 139, 141

G

Gallbladder, 88
Gallstones, 90
Gastric glands, 83
Gastroenteritis, 5
Gastrointestinal disturbances,
    107
Genetics, 55
Germinal epithelium, 155
Giantism, 126
Ginger compress, 9, 34, 45,
    188
Ginger sesame oil, 188
Glaucoma, 129, 164
Glucagon, 123, 130
Glucose, 123, 132, 133
Glycogen, 93
Glycosuria, 129
Go-Gyo, 75
Go-Koku, 72
Goiter, 126
Gomasio, 31, 188
Gonads, 120, 124, 129

Gonorrhea, 161
Grains, cereal, 29, 30, 32
Grandparents, 52, 53, 54
Granulocytes, 104, 105
Graves' disease, 126
Gross, Martin, 7
Ground beef plaster, 99
Gull's disease, 126
Gums, 169
Gynecology, 6

H

Habits, 57
Hair, 61, 171
Hair, body, 62
Hair spiral, 65, 143
Halitosis, 102
Handwriting, 64
Hara, 66, 83, 105, 145, 175
Haramaki, 83
Harelip, 59
Hay fever, 5, 35, 101
Head, 163
Headaches, 71
Headaches, migraine, 150
Hearing, impaired, 36
Heart, 29, 38, 39, 59, 72,
    111, 112, 113
Heaven's force, 20, 66, 67,
    120, 121, 143
Hematin, 103
Hemoglobin, 103, 106
Hemolytic reaction, 109
Hemophilia, 9, 108
Hemophilus ducreyi, 161
Hemorrhage, cerebral, 112,
Hemorrhoids, 93
Hermatology, 9
Hernia, 9, 92
Hernia, 9, 92
Hiccough, 102
Hijiki, 30, 92, 172
Hip bath, 159, 188
Honey, 32, 94
Hookworms, 86
Hodgkin's disease, 114
Hormones, 119–127
Hydrochloric acid, 83, 110
Hydrocele, 155
Hyperglycemia, 129
Hyperinsulinism, 127, 132, 133
Hypertension, 5, 112
Hypocalcemic tetany, 5
Hypoglycemia, 132

Hypophysis cerebri, 121
Hypotension, 112
Hysterectomy, 7, 10

I

I Ching, 169
Imagination 139
Imbalance, 33
Immunization factors, 114
Implantation, 157, 173, 175
Impotency, 38, 153
Indecision, 86
Infant care, 179–184
Infections disease, 26
Inferior vena cava, 143
Internal medicine, 6, 7
Insulin, 123, 127, 129, 130,
    132, 133
Intestines, 35, 61, 65, 84, 85,
    90, 91, 123, 124, 125
Intestinal villi, *see* Villi
Intrinsic factor, 107
Iodine, 126
Irish moss, 30
Islets of Langerhans, 123,
    129, 130, 132
Itching, 89

J

Jaundice, 89
Jejunum, 85
Jesus, 28, 55
Ji-So, 50

K

Kan-Jin, 88
Kan-Shaku, 88
Kass, Dr. Edward, 117
Ketone bodies, 129
Ki, 78, 143
Ki-Kai, 83
Kidneys, 35, 37, 60, 72, 123
Kikuchi, Tomio, 12
Koi-Koku, 162
Kombu (Kelp), 30, 31, 160, 172
Kuzu (Kudzu) drink, 188

L

Labor, 176–179
Lactation, 33
Lao Tsu, 55

Large intestine, 41, 42, 69, 72
Larynx, 95
Legs, 34, 91, 184
Lens, 163
Leucocytes, 104
Leukemia, 7, 9, 104
Lips, 61, 62, 91
Liquid, 75
Liver, 60, 69, 72, 88, 89, 115
Lobules, 153
Lotus root plaster, 36, 189
LSD, 12, 140
Lunar cycle, 49, 157
Lungs, 36, 59, 72, 95, 96
Lymphatic system, 39, 40, 46, 83, 114, 115
Lymphocytes, 104, 105, 114
Lymphosarcoma, 114

M

McGovern, Senator George, 30
Macrobiotic healing, principles of 23; aim of, 19
Macrobiotic eating, standard, 29, 30
Maison Ignoramus, 11
Malaria, 107
Male reproductive system, 153
Mammary glands, 121
Mammography, 7
Maple syrup, 32, 94
Marijuana, 12
Martial arts, 32
Massage, 70, 71
Measles, 184
Meat, 32, 90
Medications, 32, 46
Medicine, modern, 8, 9, 10; preventive, 7
Meditation, 56
Memory, 56, 86, 138, 141
Meningitis, 7
Menopause, 117
Menstruation, 17, 33, 102, 127, 157–160
Mental illness, 24
Mental retardation, 174
Meridians, 65, 66, 68, 70, 72, 75–78, 119, 128
Meridian diagnosis, 69–71
Metabolism, 123, 125, 129
Midbrain, 120, 121, 137, 138
Migraine, 150
Milk, 32, 179, 180, 184

Millet, 30, 130
Minerals, 106, 123, 125
Miscarriage, 127, 135, 176
Miso, 30
Mochi, 87, 184
Mohammed, 28
Molars, 169, 170
Moles, 62
Mongolism, 7
Monocytes, 104, 105
Monosaccharides, 93
Monosodium glutamate (MSG), 41
Moon, full and new, 49
Morning sickness, 173
Moustache, 62
Moxa, 36, 38
Mu tea, 30
Mucus, 35, 89
Mugwort, 87
Multiple sclerosis, 128, 152
Mumps, 185
Muscle spasms, 126
Mustard, 35, 36
Mycobacterium tuberculosis, 99
Mydexedema, 126
Myopia, 10

N

Nakamura. Ave, 12
Natural applications, 187
Natural birth, 12
Navel, 79
Nearsightedness, 71, 165
Necrotizing enterocolitis, 5
Neisseria gonorrhoeae, 161
Neonatal hypothyroidism, 5
Neonatal period, 182
Nervous system, 25, 54, 83, 135, 142
Neurophils, 104, 105
New England Journal of Medicine, 117
Nishime, 147
Noradrenalin, 123
Nori, 30
Nose, 39, 59, 101, 102, 113
Nut butters, 91
Nutrition, scientific, 9
Nuts, roasted, 30

O

OB-GYN, 6, 7

Obesity, 5
Obstetrics, 6
Odor, body, 9, 64
Ohsawa, George, 11, 12, 17, 18
Oil, 30, 112, 189
Optic nerve, 163, 164
Oranges, 32
Order of the universe, principles of, 193
Organ diseases, 25
Organs, yin and yang, 40, 41
Orinase, 130
Oriental medicine, 49, 58, 70, 75, 79, 85
Orthosympathetic nerves, 123, 135, 137
Osteitis fibrosa, 126
Ovarian cysts, 38, 46
Ovaries, 124, 125, 145, 146, 155, 156, 157
Overeating, 43
Ovum, 156, 173

P

Pains, 25
Plate, 102
Palm healing, 12, 181
Palms, lines on, 53
Pancreas, 60, 120, 123, 125, 127, 129, 130
Pap smear, 7
Paralysis, 7, 145
Parasympathetic nerves, 123, 135, 137, 140
Parathyroid glands, 120, 122, 125, 126, 128
Parents, 31, 52
Parkinson's disease, 149
Parturition, 176
Pediatrics, 5, 6, 7
Penicillin, 7
Penis, 67, 121, 146
Pepsin, 83, 87
Peristalsis, 135
Perspiration, 33
PH factor, 83, 112
Pharynx, 102
Phonocardiography, 7,
Pickles, quick, 34
Pill, The, 7
Pimples, 39, 59, 60, 127
Pinworms, 86
Pituitary cachexia, 126
Pituitary gland, 120, 121, 124, 126, 128

PKU testing, 7
Placenta, 120, 124, 177
Plasma, 75, 103
"Plasma Lipids and Lipoproteins in Vegetarians," 117
Pleura, 95
Pleurisy, 101
Pneumonia, 5, 7, 9, 97–99
Polio, 50
Pollen, 35, 101
Polysaccharides, 93
Postmenopausal hormones, 7
Pregnancy, 120, 124, 157, 173–176
Premature birth, 176
Pressure-points, 35, 71
Primary channel, 66, 143, 175
Principles of the order of the universe, 193
Progesterone, 124, 125, 127, 157
Protein, 85, 123, 180
Psoriasis, 42
Psychiatry, 7
Psychology, 24
Psycho-surgery, 7
Puberty, 124, 182
Pulmonary arteries and veins, 95
Pulse, 77, 78
Putrefaction, 32, 65, 85

R

Radiation, 35
Ranshio, 189
Rectum, 42
Rei-So, 55
Renal circuit, 110
Renal threshold, 129
Reproductive system, 61, 153
Respiration, 33, 95
Retardation, mental, 174
Rete testis, 154
Retina, 163
Retroversion of uterus, 159
Rh factor, 108
Ribcage, 71, 72
Rice, brown, 184
Rice, refined, 41
RNA, 141
Rockefeller Institute, 18

S

Saccharine, 42

Sacks, Dr. Frank, 117
Sacral nerves, 136
Salad, 30, 34
Saliva, 83, 120, 168
Salt, 30, 32
Salt bancha tea, 189
Salt pack, 45, 189
Salt water, 189
San-In-Ko, 38, 72
San-Ri, 74
Scallion juice, 188
Schizophrenia, 86
Schweitzer, Albert, 55
Scurvy, 169
Sebaceous gland, 171
Secretin, 123
Seeds, 30, 87
Seitan, 147
Sesame oil application, 35, 163
Sex, 66, 67, 105, 124, 127
Sexual hormones, 120
Sexual organs, 38, 188
Shiatsu massage, 12
Shin, 49
Shintoism, 17
Shio-kombu, 162
Shivering, 34
Shoku-Shin, 71
Showers, 31, 93
Silver nitrate, 10
Sinuses, 35
Skin, 34, 62, 67, 80
Skin wash, 34
Sleeping pills, 174
Sleepwalking, 57
Smoking, 96, 97
Sneezing, 101
Snoring, 103
So, 49
So-So, 56
Soba, 87
Social disharmony, 24
Socrates, 55
Sodium bicarbonate, 110
Sodium chloride, 110
Soft drinks, 32
Solar system, 142
Soup, miso or tamari, 30
Space, 141
Speech, 102
Sperm, 121, 153, 154
Spine, 135
Spiritual channel, 119, 143, 145
Spiritual influence, 55, 56

Spleen, 60, 69, 74, 114
Sports, 32
Stomach, 41, 59, 87, 88
Stroke, 112
Sugar, 32, 94, 129
Sugar Blues, 94
Sun baths, 100
Surgery, 6, 7, 35
Suribachi, 31, 45, 46, 184
Sweating, abnormal, 34
Sweet brown rice, 87, 184
Swine flu vaccine, 7
Symptoms, 80
Synthetic fibers, 35; also see Clothing
Syphilis, 161
Szasz, Thomas, 7

T

Tai-kyo, 174
Tamari bancha tea, 190
Tamari soy sauce, 30, 31, 91
Tampon preparation, 160
Taoism, 17
Tapeworms, 86
Taro potato (albi) plaster, 45, 190
Tea, commercially produced, 32
Teeth, 26, 27, 54, 71, 168, 183
Tekka, 31
Ten-So, 49
Testis, 124, 125, 127, 146, 153
Testosterone, 124
Tetany, 126
Thermography, 7
Thinking, 33, 139
Thoracic cavity, 95
Thoracoplasty, 100
Threadworms, 86
Throat, 120
Thrombosis, cerebral, 112
Thymus, 114
Thyroid gland, 120, 121, 125, 126, 128
Thyroxin, 122, 125, 126
Time, 50, 141
Tiredness, 24
Tofu plaster, 190
Tongue, 65, 120, 145
Tonsillectomy, 7, 39, 46, 115, 146
Tonsils, 115, 145, 146
Toothache, 71

Trachea, 95, 97
Tranquilizers, 7, 174
Transformations, five, 75, 77
Transmutation, 106
Transverse colon, 42
Treponema pallidum, 161
Triple Heater, 75, 77
Tuberculosis, 99, 100
Tumors, fibroid, 46
Tunica albuginea, 153

U

Ulcers, 88
Umbilical cord, 178
Umeboshi plum, juice of, 91, 171
Umeboshi plum, pits, baked, 190
Umeboshi plums, 31, 91, 190
Ume-sho-bancha, 190
Ume-sho-kuzu, 190
Universal consciousness, 142, 182
Universe, 29, 141
Universe, seven principles of, 193, twelve laws of, 193
Urination, 34, 37, 79, 135
Uterine cysts, 159, 160
Uterus, 146, 155, 156, 157, 160, 177

Uvula, 67, 120, 146

V

Vaccination, 23
Vagina, 38, 67, 159, 160
Vasectomy, 7
Vedanta, 17
Vegetables, 30, 32, 107
Venereal disease, 161, 162
Vertebrae, 54, 55, 135
Vibrations, 55, 56, 138, 141
Villi, 40, 67, 85, 105
Vinegar, 32
Vision, double, 71
Vision, future, 139, 141
Visual diagnosis, 58
Vitality, lack of, 105
Vitamins, 65, 107
Vocal cords, 95, 102
Voice, 64, 102

W

Wakame, 31, 172
Water molecule, 119
Waves, alpha and beta, 56
Way of life, 81
Whipworms, 86
Whooping cough, 100
Windpipe, 95

Wisdom teeth, 27
Whole wheat, 30
Wool, 35; *also see* Clothing
Worms, 86; *also see* name of worm

X

X-ray, 7

Y

Yamamoto, Shizuko, 12
Yamazaki, Junsei, 12
Yasuhara, Roland, 12
Yin and yang, 18, 20, 193, 194
Yin and yang constitutions, 58
Yin and yang foods, 32
Yin and yang transformations, 77
Yoga, 32
Yoghurt, 32
Yoshimi, Clim, 12
Yu-Sen, 72

Z

Zen, 28
Ziskind, Jay, 7
Zucchini, 32